CONTENTS

3

INTRODUCTION

Nowadays there are a lot of kitchen appliances promising wonderful things, but people aren't aware that air fryers are exactly the ones that are worth the money spent to buy them.

Buying an air fryer is the way to adopt a healthy lifestyle and to fight against chronic diseases in the long term.

The Air fryer is a type of appliance that promises to function for more than one way; it can roast, bake, and grill. It has the least uses of oil, and sometimes it does not use oil at all. It provides food with the same texture and way it would be provided with the old traditional ways of frying. An air fryer is very compact, and nowadays, almost every kitchen should be equipped with an appliance like this. It also works as a conventional oven and microwave at the same time.

There is a lot of debate that goes on whether it is worth investing the money and if it stands out for what it promises. Air fryers would save people their time and health. There are a lot of things that people are not aware of air fryers. So, let's go on.

What Is An Air Fryer And How To Use It For Cooking?

An Air fryer is a kitchen appliance that really helps in cooking. It circulates hot air around the food using a Convection mechanism. Convection is heat transfer because of the movement of molecules between fluids. In the past, a lot of houses didn't have an air fryer and used a Convection oven, which is an oven that has fans and circulates heat around the food. It has a convection mechanism that helps the food to cook faster.

Convection oven was used for industrial applications. An air fryer is a smaller version of the oven. It has a mechanical fan, which is a powerful machine that helps to create a flow. It also has a rotating arrangement of blades that act as air. It circulates hot air around the food at a very high speed and helps in cooking the food. It produces a Crusty Brown layer over the top of it. It cooks food in less oil or no oil, and it is a very healthy lifestyle adaptation. With more knowledge of a healthy lifestyle in today's era, people are trying to adapt to air fryers. The air fryer is used for a lot of purposes, whether it is cooking or heating the food.

A lot of people have completely decided to replace microwaves and conventional ovens with a fryer. It is a very healthy alternative for them. The traditional frying methods submerge food into hot oil at a very high temperature. An air fryer is completely different than that. In an air fryer, a thin layer of oil on the food is applied and circulated on at least two hundred degrees Celsius. The heat supplies, the reaction initiate and this makes possible to make the food caramelize or turn brown. Many of the Air fryers have temperature and time adjustment. It helps in precise cooking. It makes it easier to know for how long and at what temperature it would be ready. As soon as the airstrikes, the food starts to caramelize or turn brown.

Today people are always looking for the latest cooking appliances. That's the demand of today's era. Among every other appliance, an air fryer is the one that people want. An air fryer is like an oven because it also bakes and roasts but it is very compact and smaller compared to other ovens. The difference is also that the heating elements that are located on the top.

They're also accompanied by a powerful fan or blade that rotates the air. It makes the food Crispier and is ready in almost no time because of the combination of the concentrated heat source and the placement of the fan.

The air fryer has a great clean up system. That consists of the fryer basket and racks that are dishwasher safe. The ones that are not dishwashers safe can be easily done with a good dish brush.

The air fried food is very comparable to the results of a different oven. It makes food crispy on the outside and juicy on the inside. It only needs a tiny amount of oil and sometimes doesn't need oil at all, depending on what you are actually cooking. It's a very healthy alternative for people trying to adopt a healthy lifestyle, trying to omit oil from life. That's because it comes into use by one or two tablespoons of oil and a little seasoning. For this reason, this appliance reduces the risk of chronic disease and tends to provide long-term health benefits.

Cooking food in the air fryer is very easy and fast to use, and it can be used to heat or cook both quick fresh foods and frozen foods. Most of the meals do not need oil because they are juicy by themselves. What you have to do is to season with salt or your favorite Herbs and Spices. You should use dry Seasoning because when there is less moisture, it helps to keep the food crispy. If you want to add any sort of sauce, you should wait until there are only one to two minutes left and then add to It, so the food stays crispy and does not end soggy with time.

Who Should Use An Air Fryer?

The air fryer can be used by anyone:

• THE WEIGHT WATCHER: People that are very weight conscious can cook food with minimal oil or no oil at all. Still, the food will taste delicious, and they can have healthy low-fat food.

• THE BUSY PARENT: Parents are very busy and have a lot of house chores to do. They also have to take care after the toddlers or the children if they are working. They don't have enough time to cook. It is the actual experience of hands-free cooking. They can attend any other chores because the air fryer is an automatic appliance.

• THE ELDERLY: It is very easy to use because it hasn't any complicated buttons to press. It is a fuss-free air fryer. Elderly people having difficulty in cooking can take pre-cooked meals. They are easy to prepare in an air fryer because it's very easy to use.

• THE STUDENTS/SINGLES: People who study or live alone, they do not have enough time to cook food. So with an air fryer, they can cook their favorite small meals any day in a frame because it is very convenient to use.

• KIDS: Kids are not allowed to go to the kitchen because they can burn down the house. With an air fryer, they can cook delicious meals without any danger.

Air fryer meal is similar to what is cooked in a conventional oven, but it only cooks faster and with less oil. There is no certain age limit for who should consume air fryer meals. It is a healthy lifestyle that can be adopted by people of any age. Life with an air fryer is very healthy, and this way, people can enjoy foods with nobility. French fries, chicken wings and beef, if cooked with an air fryer, can be enjoyed by people of every age because because there is no oil consumption that adds to the fat.

People who are on a diet are trying to omit oil from their life because it leads to chronic diseases. The best alternative is the air fryer. It is one of the best ways through which they can eat and enjoy. It benefits a lot and actually outweighs the risk of eating food that is having a lot of calories.

Instead of completely submerging the food in oil, the air fryer requires a tablespoon of oil to achieve the food that has a similar taste and texture to Deep fried food. It also helps to cut down the fat content because some foods are actually very high. Instead of this requires less fat than traditional deep fryers. This is the difference: it uses up to 50 times less oil that is used in a normal oven. Oil is absorbed by the food as a larger fraction significant above the fat content of the food. It has a great impact on health as a higher intake of fried food from vegetable oil. The people who want to save them from any sort of chronic disease can use an air fryer. It is the best way they can enjoy their food without getting the risk of it.

An air fryer also helps in a weight loss of people who have problems with obesity and their trying to lose weight. So those people can actually switch to air fryers because it may help in weight loss. People trying to trim the waistline and trying to lose inches can swap meals because it is a good place to start. Gym freaks or fitness freaks can opt Air fryer because air fryer foods are low in fat. It is also a good way to cut calories.

Not all machines are age-friendly, but the air is a type of machine that can be used by people of any age. The numerous numbers of meals can be made in the air fryer can be enjoyed by kids or by elders. There is no certain age; it is beneficial to everyone. That is one of the biggest pros of an air fryer. A child who wants to enjoy the favorite food can put it in the air fryer and press the button, and it will be cooked in no time. It is all a game of buttons.

Benefits Of Air Fryer

The evidence that air fryer has a lot of benefits can be proven by the benefits listed down below:

1. LOW-FAT COOKER: Cooking in air fryer people don't have to add any oil when frying Frozen Food. All they need to do is take it out from the freezer and put it in the air fryer and adjust the time. Temperature and no oil is actually needed for meals. The rapid circulating system actually cooks food from all angles. It is a very low-fat way of cooking, and the excess fat from the meals are cut down from it.

2. AUTOMATIC COOKER: it is a very simple process because two types of air fryer are available in the market. One is with a steering pedal, and the other one is the bowl method. People are so busy carrying out different Life chores. They don't get the time to stand in front of the stove to keep on monitoring the cooking process. But with the automatic cooker, all you have to do is place a portion of food into the air fryer and let it cook by itself. In designated times, you don't have to stand in the kitchen. In that period of time, you can carry out different activities. This automatic cooker is not only splatter-free, it olso helps you to not spread oil into the kitchen.

3. IT IS FUSS FREE: It is simple to use because it only has a button to press. All you have to do is to set the timer and the temperature, and the meal is ready as soon as the timer goes off. Some of the air fryers also come with fixed temperature settings, which make it easier to cook.

They also come with research programs. If you are unaware you can use a preset with a particular cooking time. All you have to do is to press the button, and the meal that you are trying to cook will be cooked without any fuss. It is very easy to cook, and it is not hectic and also very fuss-free.

4. IT IS FAST AND CONVENIENT: it is a very fast and convenient way to cook. The compact air fryer actually does not need to be preheated. It is needed in the conventional oven. The food cooked is actually enclosed in the fryer cooker. So, there is no mess to clean up like there is no idea for waiting, and there is no oil all the way on the stove. So people can actually use air fryers because they are quick and convenient. We can also use leftover food, and most of them only need like about 5-7 minutes to reheat, and the crispy food is ready. A cooker is actually very practical when it comes to cooking as compared to a Convection oven. People who are trying to cook small portions of food, they just turn on the air fryer. It is very cheap and qick. Cooking is not only very handy and convenient, but also safe and healthy.

5. SAFE TO USE: Air fryers come with a lot of safety features. It also has an auto-shutdown feature when the cooking is partially completed. This is very beneficial. It reduces the risk of overheating. It also prevents the food from Burning down. The air fryer also has a non-slip field that minimizes the risk of the machine sliding down the counter. The machine also saves the food from burning, keeping the kitchen safe. The close system provides spilling free cooking experience. There is no way the oil can splash out. These machines are also certified. This means that they're widely accepted for safety standards. This way, everybody can cook food on wheels in the air fryer without elder help. Elders can make it without any fuss, and all they need is the air fryer.

6. IT IS A MULTI TASKER COOKER: Air Fryer is a machine that does not only fry but also bakes roast and grills. It is a highly versatile appliance. For this reason it is also known as a multi-cooker hot air fryer. It has skills that no oven or hot grill can have in one compact machine. We can use the air fryer for breakfast, lunch and dinner, even for the snacks. In today's world, when everything is so fast-paced, everything is Technology related. This High versatile machine makes the whole cooking process convenient. It is very easy for managing people who don't like cooking and also serves healthy fat free meals in no time.

7. EASY TO CLEAN: Air fryers are very easy to clean. All the parts of the Fryer are removable and also dishwasher-safe. So, even if people don't have a dishwasher, they can actually submerge it in water and then gently rub a sponge. This removes any sort of bits and pieces that might be stuck on the cooking surface. So it is very easy to clean compared to other machines that actually create a fuss while cleaning.

8. SAVES THE BUDGET OF COOKING OIL: Since hardly any oil is used in air fryers, you will save money for sure. It is very budget-friendly.

9. IT IS HEALTHIER WAY OF COOKING: The air fryer offers healthy dishes as compared to other fryers. It is designed specifically to function without any failures. It produces food with 80% less fat, and it can also help to lose weight.

People have been trying to get rid of it. It can be very difficult for people to let go of the fried food. In this case they can keep eating theyr favourite fried food or try to roast it as an alternative. After all it is the perfect way that anybody is looking for to switch to a healthy lifestyle.

10. FOOD SEPARATOR: The air fryer is supplied with the food separator. That enables us to prepare multiple healthy meals at once. The separator makes it very quick and easy to make meal combinations. Thanks to this simple feature, you can cook different ingredients at the same time with similar temperature settings saving your time.

11. AIR FILTER: Many air fryers have an integrated air filter. It helps to remove any sort of unwanted smell that is being spread around the house.

12. COST EFFECTIVE: I have no doubt to confirm that an air fryer is a very cost-effective appliance. It cost moderately in the market and gives out a lot of features in a single appliance, so it is very budget-friendly. Nowadays there are a lot of companies that are selling and manufacturing air fryers, which is an advantage for the buyers, giving the opportunity to purchase according to their budget.

APPETIZERS AND SIDE DISHES

1. Grandma's Chicken Thighs

Servings: 2
Cooking Time: 30 Minutes
Ingredients:
- 1 pound chicken thighs
- ½ tsp salt
- ¼ tsp black pepper
- ¼ tsp garlic powder

Directions:
1. Season the thighs with salt, pepper, and garlic powder. Arrange thighs, skin side down, on the Air Fryer basket and fit in the baking tray. Cook until golden brown, about 20 minutes at 350 F on Bake function. Serve immediately.

2. Baked Potatoes With Yogurt And Chives

Servings:4
Cooking Time: 35 Minutes
Ingredients:
- 4 (7-ounce / 198-g) russet potatoes, rinsed
- Olive oil spray
- ½ teaspoon kosher salt, divided
- ½ cup 2% plain Greek yogurt
- ¼ cup minced fresh chives
- Freshly ground black pepper, to taste

Directions:
1. Pat the potatoes dry and pierce them all over with a fork. Spritz the potatoes with olive oil spray. Sprinkle with ¼ teaspoon of the salt.
2. Transfer the potatoes to the baking pan.
3. Slide the baking pan into Rack Position 1, select Convection Bake, set temperature to 400ºF (205ºC), and set time to 35 minutes.
4. When cooking is complete, the potatoes should be fork-tender. Remove from the oven and split open the potatoes. Top with the yogurt, chives, the remaining ¼ teaspoon of salt, and finish with the black pepper. Serve immediately.

3. Creamy Broccoli Casserole

Servings: 6
Cooking Time: 30 Minutes
Ingredients:
- 16 oz frozen broccoli florets, defrosted and drained
- 1/2 tsp onion powder
- 10.5 oz can cream of mushroom soup
- 1 cup cheddar cheese, shredded
- 1/3 cup almond milk
- For topping:
- 1 tbsp butter, melted
- 1/2 cup cracker crumbs

Directions:
1. Fit the oven with the rack in position
2. Add all ingredients except topping ingredients into the 1.5-qt casserole dish.
3. In a small bowl, mix together cracker crumbs and melted butter and sprinkle over the casserole dish mixture.
4. Set to bake at 350 F for 35 minutes. After 5 minutes place the casserole dish in the preheated oven.
5. Serve and enjoy.
- **Nutrition Info:** Calories 203 Fat 13.5 g Carbohydrates 11.9 g Sugar 3.6 g Protein 6.9 g Cholesterol 26 mg

4. Easy Parsnip Fries

Servings: 3
Cooking Time: 15 Minutes
Ingredients:
- 4 parsnips, sliced
- ¼ cup flour
- ¼ cup olive oil
- ¼ cup water
- A pinch of salt

Directions:
1. Preheat on Air Fry function to 390 F. In a bowl, add the flour, olive oil, water, and parsnips; mix to coat. Line the fries in the greased Air Fryer basket and fit in the baking tray. Cook for 15 minutes. Serve with yogurt and garlic dip.

5. Baked Paprika Sweet Potatoes

Servings: 4
Cooking Time: 20 Minutes
Ingredients:
- 3 sweet potatoes, peel and cut into 1/2-inch pieces
- 2 tbsp olive oil
- 1/2 tsp pepper
- 2 tsp smoked paprika
- 1 tsp garlic salt

Directions:
1. Fit the oven with the rack in position
2. Add sweet potatoes, paprika, oil, pepper, and salt into the mixing bowl and toss well.
3. Spread sweet potatoes in baking pan.
4. Set to bake at 425 F for 25 minutes. After 5 minutes place the baking pan in the preheated oven.
5. Serve and enjoy.
- **Nutrition Info:** Calories 155 Fat 7.3 g Carbohydrates 22.2 g Sugar 0.7 g Protein 1.5 g Cholesterol 0 mg

6. Garlic Potato Chips

Servings: 3
Cooking Time: 30 Minutes + Marinating Time
Ingredients:

- 3 whole potatoes, cut into thin slices
- ¼ cup olive oil
- 1 tbsp garlic
- ½ cup cream
- 2 tbsp rosemary

Directions:
1. Preheat on Air Fry function to 390 F. In a bowl, add oil, garlic, and salt to form a marinade. Stir in the potatoes. Allow sitting for 30 minutes.
2. Lay the potato slices onto the Air Fryer basket and fit in the baking tray. Cook for 20 minutes. After 10 minutes, give the chips a turn. When readt, sprinkle with rosemary and serve.

7. Lemon Parmesan And Peas Risotto

Servings: 6
Cooking Time: 17 Minutes
Ingredients:
- 2 tablespoons butter
- 1½ cup rice
- 1 yellow onion, peeled and chopped
- 1 tablespoon extra-virgin olive oil
- 1 teaspoon lemon zest, grated
- 3½ cups chicken stock
- 2 tablespoons lemon juice
- 2 tablespoons parsley, diced
- 2 tablespoons Parmesan cheese, finely grated
- Salt and ground black pepper, to taste
- 1½ cup peas

Directions:
1. Put the Instant Pot in the sauté mode, add 1 tablespoon of butter and oil and heat them. Add the onion, mix and cook for 5 minutes.
2. Add the rice, mix and cook for another 3 minutes. Add 3 cups of broth and lemon juice, mix, cover and cook for 5 minutes on rice.
3. Release the pressure, put the Instant Pot in manual mode, add the peas and the rest of the broth, stir and cook for 2 minutes.
4. Add the cheese, parsley, remaining butter, lemon zest, salt and pepper to taste and mix. Divide between plates and serve.
- **Nutrition Info:** Calories: 140, Fat: 1.5, Fiber: 1, Carbohydrate: 27, Proteins: 5

8. Cheddar Cheese Cauliflower Casserole

Servings: 8
Cooking Time: 35 Minutes
Ingredients:
- 4 cups cauliflower florets
- 1 1/2 cups cheddar cheese, shredded
- 1 cup sour cream
- 4 bacon slices, cooked and crumbled
- 3 green onions, chopped

Directions:

1. Fit the oven with the rack in position
2. Boil water in a large pot. Add cauliflower in boiling water and cook for 8-10 minutes or until tender. Drain well.
3. Transfer cauliflower in a large bowl.
4. Add half bacon, half green onion, 1 cup cheese, and sour cream in cauliflower bowl and mix well.
5. Transfer mixture into a greased baking dish and sprinkle with remaining cheese.
6. Set to bake at 350 F for 30 minutes. After 5 minutes place the baking dish in the preheated oven.
7. Garnish with remaining green onion and bacon.
8. Serve and enjoy.
- **Nutrition Info:** Calories 213 Fat 17.1 g Carbohydrates 4.7 g Sugar 1.5 g Protein 10.8 g Cholesterol 45 mg

9. Honey Corn Muffins

Servings: 8
Cooking Time: 20 Minutes
Ingredients:
- 2 eggs
- 1/2 cup sugar
- 1 1/4 cups self-rising flour
- 3/4 cup yellow cornmeal
- 1/2 cup butter, melted
- 3/4 cup buttermilk
- 1 tbsp honey

Directions:
1. Fit the oven with the rack in position
2. Spray 8-cups muffin tin with cooking spray and set aside.
3. In a large bowl, mix together cornmeal, sugar, and flour.
4. In a separate bowl, whisk the eggs with buttermilk and honey until well combined.
5. Slowly add egg mixture and melted butter to the cornmeal mixture and stir until just mixed.
6. Spoon batter into the prepared muffin tin.
7. Set to bake at 350 F for 25 minutes. After 5 minutes place muffin tin in the preheated oven.
8. Serve and enjoy.
- **Nutrition Info:** Calories 294 Fat 13.4 g Carbohydrates 39.6 g Sugar 16 g Protein 5.2 g Cholesterol 72 mg

10. Yogurt Masala Cashew

Servings: 2
Cooking Time: 25 Minutes
Ingredients:
- 8 oz Greek yogurt
- 2 tbsp mango powder
- 8¾ oz cashew nuts
- Salt and black pepper to taste

- 1 tsp coriander powder
- ½ tsp masala powder
- ½ tsp black pepper powder

Directions:
1. Preheat on Air Fry function to 350 F. In a bowl, mix all powders, salt, and pepper. Add in cashews and toss to coat thoroughly. Place the cashews in your Air Fryer baking pan and cook for 15 minutes, shaking every 5 minutes. Serve.

11. Cabbage Wedges With Parmesan

Servings: 4
Cooking Time: 30 Minutes
Ingredients:
- ½ head of cabbage, cut into 4 wedges
- 4 tbsp butter, melted
- 2 cups Parmesan cheese, grated
- Salt and black pepper to taste
- 1 tsp smoked paprika

Directions:
1. Preheat on Air Fry function to 330 F. Line a baking sheet with parchment paper. Brush the cabbage wedges with the butter. Season with salt and pepper.
2. Coat cabbage with Parmesan cheese and arrange on the baking pan; sprinkle with paprika. Cook for 15 minutes, flip, and cook for an additional 10 minutes. Serve with yogurt dip.

12. Roasted Beets With Grapefruit Glaze

Servings: 5
Cooking Time: 10 Minutes
Ingredients:
- 3 pounds beets
- 1 cup fresh-squeezed grapefruit juice (approximately 2 medium grapefruits)
- 1 tablespoon rice vinegar
- 3 scant tablespoons pure maple syrup
- 1 tablespoon corn starch

Directions:
1. Start by preheating toaster oven to 450°F. Place beets in a roasting pan and sprinkle with water.
2. Roast beets until soft enough to be pierced with a fork, at least 40 minutes.
3. Remove beets and allow to cool until you can handle them.
4. Peel skin off beets and thinly slice.
5. Mix together grapefruit juice, syrup, and vinegar in a small bowl.
6. Pour corn starch into a medium sauce pan and slowly add grapefruit mixture. Stir together until there are no clumps.
7. Heat sauce to a light boil then reduce heat and simmer for 5 minutes, stirring often.
8. Drizzle glaze over beets and serve.

- **Nutrition Info:** Calories: 175, Sodium: 211 mg, Dietary Fiber: 6.0 g, Total Fat: 0.6 g, Total Carbs: 40.7 g, Protein: 4.9 g.

13. Garlic Brussels Sprouts

Servings:4
Cooking Time: 25 Minutes
Ingredients:
- 1 pound Brussels sprouts
- 1 garlic clove, minced
- 2 tbsp olive oil
- Salt and black pepper to taste

Directions:
1. Wash the Brussels sprouts thoroughly under cold water and trim off the outer leaves, keeping only the head of the sprouts. In a bowl, mix olive oil and garlic. Season with salt and pepper.
2. Add in the prepared sprouts let rest for 5 minutes. Place the coated sprouts in the frying basket. Select AirFry function, adjust the temperature to 380 F, and press Start. Cook for 15 minutes.

14. Savory Cod Fingers

Servings:3
Cooking Time: 25 Minutes
Ingredients:
- 2 cups flour
- 1 tsp seafood seasoning
- 2 whole eggs, beaten
- 1 cup cornmeal
- 1 pound cod fillets, cut into fingers
- 2 tbsp milk
- 2 eggs, beaten
- 1 cup breadcrumbs

Directions:
1. Preheat on Air Fryer function to 400 F. In a bowl, mix beaten eggs with milk. In a separate bowl, mix flour, cornmeal, and seafood seasoning. In a third bowl, pour the breadcrumbs.
2. Dip cod fingers in the flour mixture, followed by a dip in the egg mixture and finally coat with breadcrumbs. Place the fingers in the frying basket and Press Start. AirFry for 10 minutes.

15. Sausage Mushroom Caps(2)

Servings: 2
Cooking Time: 20 Minutes
Ingredients:
- ½ lb. Italian sausage
- 6 large Portobello mushroom caps
- ¼ cup grated Parmesan cheese.
- ¼ cup chopped onion
- 2 tbsp. blanched finely ground almond flour
- 1 tsp. minced fresh garlic

Directions:

1. Use a spoon to hollow out each mushroom cap, reserving scrapings.
2. In a medium skillet over medium heat, brown the sausage about 10 minutes or until fully cooked and no pink remains. Drain and then add reserved mushroom scrapings, onion, almond flour, Parmesan and garlic.
3. Gently fold ingredients together and continue cooking an additional minute, then remove from heat
4. Evenly spoon the mixture into mushroom caps and place the caps into a 6-inch round pan. Place pan into the air fryer basket
5. Adjust the temperature to 375 Degrees F and set the timer for 8 minutes. When finished cooking, the tops will be browned and bubbling. Serve warm.
- **Nutrition Info:** Calories: 404; Protein: 24.3g; Fiber: 4.5g; Fat: 25.8g; Carbs: 18.2g

16. Crispy Eggplant Fries

Servings: 2
Cooking Time: 20 Minutes
Ingredients:
- 1 eggplant, sliced
- 1 tsp olive oil
- 1 tsp soy sauce
- Salt to taste

Directions:
1. Preheat on Air Fry function to 400 F. Make a marinade of 1 tsp oil, soy sauce, and salt. Mix well. Add in the eggplant slices and let stand for 5 minutes. Place the prepared eggplant slices in the cooking basket and fit in the baking tray. Cook for 8 minutes. Serve warm.

17. Broiled Prosciutto-wrapped Pears

Servings: 8
Cooking Time: 6 Minutes
Ingredients:
- 2 large, ripe Anjou pears
- 4 thin slices Parma prosciutto
- 2 teaspoons aged balsamic vinegar

Directions:
1. Peel the pears. Slice into 8 wedges and cut out the core from each wedge.
2. Cut the prosciutto into 8 long strips. Wrap each pear wedge with a strip of prosciutto. Place the wrapped pears in the air fryer basket.
3. Put the air fryer basket on the baking pan and slide into Rack Position 2, select Convection Broil, set temperature to High and set time to 6 minutes.
4. After 2 or 3 minutes, check the pears. The pears should be turned over if the prosciutto is beginning to crisp up and

brown. Return to the oven and continue cooking.
5. When cooking is complete, remove from the oven. Drizzle the pears with the balsamic vinegar and serve warm.

18. Parmesan Cauliflower

Servings: 5 Cups
Cooking Time: 15 Minutes
Ingredients:
- 8 cups small cauliflower florets (about 1¼ pounds / 567 g)
- 3 tablespoons olive oil
- 1 teaspoon garlic powder
- ½ teaspoon salt
- ½ teaspoon turmeric
- ¼ cup shredded Parmesan cheese

Directions:
1. In a bowl, combine the cauliflower florets, olive oil, garlic powder, salt, and turmeric and toss to coat. Transfer to the air fryer basket.
2. Put the air fryer basket on the baking pan and slide into Rack Position 2, select Air Fry, set temperature to 390ºF (199ºC), and set time to 15 minutes.
3. After 5 minutes, remove from the oven and stir the cauliflower florets. Return to the oven and continue cooking.
4. After 6 minutes, remove from the oven and stir the cauliflower. Return to the oven and continue cooking for 4 minutes. The cauliflower florets should be crisp-tender.
5. When cooking is complete, remove from the oven to a plate. Sprinkle with the shredded Parmesan cheese and toss well. Serve warm.

19. Rosemary Potatoes

Servings:4
Cooking Time: 35 Minutes
Ingredients:
- 1 ½ pounds potatoes, halved
- 2 tbsp olive oil
- 3 garlic cloves, minced
- 1 tbsp minced fresh rosemary
- Salt and black pepper to taste

Directions:
1. In a bowl, mix potatoes, olive oil, garlic, rosemary, salt, and pepper. Arrange the potatoes on the basket. Select AirFry function, adjust the temperature to 380 F, and press Start. Cook for 20-25 minutes until crispy on the outside and tender on the inside. Serve warm.

20. Baked Honey Carrots

Servings: 4
Cooking Time: 25 Minutes
Ingredients:

- 1 lb baby carrots
- 2 tbsp butter, melted
- 3 tbsp honey
- 2 tsp fresh parsley, chopped
- 1 tbsp Dijon mustard
- Pepper
- Salt

Directions:
1. Fit the oven with the rack in position
2. In a large bowl, toss carrots with Dijon mustard, honey, butter, pepper, and salt.
3. Transfer carrots in a baking dish and spread evenly.
4. Set to bake at 400 F for 30 minutes. After 5 minutes place the baking dish in the preheated oven.
5. Serve and enjoy.
- **Nutrition Info:** Calories 141 Fat 6.1 g Carbohydrates 22.6 g Sugar 18.4 g Protein 1 g Cholesterol 15 mg

21. Savory Parsley Crab Cakes

Servings: 6
Cooking Time: 20 Minutes
Ingredients:
- 1 lb crab meat, shredded
- 2 eggs, beaten
- ½ cup breadcrumbs
- ⅓ cup finely chopped green onion
- ¼ cup parsley, chopped
- 1 tbsp mayonnaise
- 1 tsp sweet chili sauce
- ½ tsp paprika
- Salt and black pepper to taste

Directions:
1. In a bowl, add crab meat, eggs, crumbs, green onion, parsley, mayo, chili sauce, paprika, salt and black pepper; mix well with your hands.
2. Shape into 6 cakes and grease them lightly with oil. Arrange them in the fryer basket without overcrowding. Fit in the baking tray and cook for 8 minutes at 400 F on Air Fry function, turning once halfway through.

22. Parmesan Dill Pickles

Servings:4
Cooking Time: 20 Minutes
Ingredients:
- 3 cups dill pickles, sliced, drained
- 2 eggs
- 2 tsp water
- 1 cup grated Parmesan cheese
- 1 ½ cups breadcrumbs, smooth
- Black pepper to taste

Directions:
1. Add the breadcrumbs and black pepper to a bowl and mix well. In another bowl, crack the eggs and beat with the water. Add the Parmesan cheese to third bowl.
2. Preheat on AirFry function to 400 F. Dredge the pickle slices in the egg mixture, then in breadcrumbs, and finally in the Parmesan cheese. Place them in the fryer oven. Press Start.AirFry for 8-10 minutes until crispy. Serve with cheese dip.

23. Roasted Curried Cauliflower

Servings: 4
Cooking Time: 35 Minutes
Ingredients:
- 1-1/2 tablespoons extra-virgin olive oil
- 1 teaspoon mustard seeds
- 1 teaspoon cumin seeds
- 3/4 teaspoon curry powder
- 3/4 teaspoon coarse salt
- 1 large head cauliflower
- Olive oil cooking spray

Directions:
1. Start by preheating toaster oven to 375°F.
2. Combine curry, mustard, cumin, and salt in a large bowl.
3. Break cauliflower into pieces and add it to the bowl.
4. Toss contents of bowl until the cauliflower is completely covered in the spice mix.
5. Coat a baking sheet in olive oil spray and lay cauliflower in a single layer over the sheet.
6. Roast for 35 minutes.
- **Nutrition Info:** Calories: 105, Sodium: 64 mg, Dietary Fiber: 5.6 g, Total Fat: 5.9 g, Total Carbs: 11.9 g, Protein: 4.5 g.

24. Cilantro Roasted Cauliflower(1)

Servings: 4
Cooking Time: 20 Minutes
Ingredients:
- 2 cups chopped cauliflower florets
- 1 medium lime
- 2 tbsp. chopped cilantro
- 2 tbsp. coconut oil; melted
- ½ tsp. garlic powder.
- 2 tsp. chili powder

Directions:
1. Take a large bowl, toss cauliflower with coconut oil. Sprinkle with chili powder and garlic powder. Place seasoned cauliflower into the air fryer basket
2. Adjust the temperature to 350 Degrees F and set the timer for 7 minutes
3. Cauliflower will be tender and begin to turn golden at the edges. Place into serving bowl. Cut the lime into quarters and squeeze juice over cauliflower. Garnish with cilantro.
- **Nutrition Info:** Calories: 73; Protein: 1g; Fiber: 1g; Fat: 5g; Carbs: 3g

25. Egg Roll Wrapped With Cabbage & Prawns

Servings: 4
Cooking Time: 50 Minutes
Ingredients:
- 2 tbsp vegetable oil
- 1-inch piece fresh ginger, grated
- 1 tbsp minced garlic
- 1 carrot, cut into strips
- ¼ cup chicken broth
- 2 tbsp reduced-sodium soy sauce
- 1 tbsp sugar
- 1 cup shredded Napa cabbage
- 1 tbsp sesame oil
- 8 cooked prawns, chopped
- 1 egg
- 8 egg roll wrappers

Directions:
1. Heat vegetable oil in a skillet over medium heat and sauté ginger and garlic for 40 seconds until fragrant. Stir in carrot and cook for another 2 minutes. Pour in chicken broth, soy sauce, and sugar and bring to a boil. Add in cabbage and let simmer until softened, about 4 minutes. Remove skillet from the heat and stir in sesame oil. Let cool for 15 minutes.
2. Strain cabbage mixture and fold in prawns. Whisk the egg in a small bowl. Fill each egg roll wrapper with prawn mixture, arranging the mixture just below the center of the wrapper. Fold the bottom part over the filling and tuck under. Fold in both sides and tightly roll-up.
3. Use the whisked egg to seal the wrapper. Repeat until all egg rolls are ready. Place the rolls into a greased frying basket, spray them with oil and fit in the baking tray. Cook for 12 minutes at 370 F on Air Fry function, turning once halfway through. Serve.

26. Mini Salmon & Cheese Quiches

Servings:15
Cooking Time: 20 Minutes
Ingredients:
- 15 mini tart cases
- 4 eggs, lightly beaten
- ½ cup heavy cream
- Salt and black pepper
- 3 oz smoked salmon
- 6 oz cream cheese, divided into 15 pieces
- 6 fresh dill

Directions:
1. Mix together eggs and heavy cream in a pourable measuring container. Arrange the tarts on the basket. Fill them with the mixture, halfway up the side and top with salmon and cream cheese. Bake for 10

minutes at 340 F on Bake function, regularly checking to avoid overcooking. Sprinkle with dill and serve chilled.

27. Healthy Green Beans

Servings: 2
Cooking Time: 10 Minutes
Ingredients:
- 8 oz green beans, trimmed and cut in half
- 1 tbsp tamari
- 1 tsp toasted sesame oil

Directions:
1. Fit the oven with the rack in position 2.
2. Add all ingredients into the large bowl and toss well.
3. Transfer green beans in the air fryer basket then place an air fryer basket in the baking pan.
4. Place a baking pan on the oven rack. Set to air fry at 400 F for 10 minutes.
5. Serve and enjoy.
- **Nutrition Info:** Calories 61 Fat 2.4 g Carbohydrates 8.6 g Sugar 1.7 g Protein 3 g Cholesterol 0 mg

28. Potatoes Au Gratin

Servings: 6
Cooking Time: 17 Minutes
Ingredients:
- ½ cup yellow onion, chopped
- 2 tablespoons butter
- 1 cup chicken stock
- 6 potatoes, peeled and sliced
- ½ cup sour cream
- Salt and ground black pepper, to taste
- 1 cup Monterey jack cheese, shredded
- For the topping:
- 3 tablespoons melted butter
- 1 cup breadcrumbs

Directions:
1. Put the Instant Pot in Saute mode, add the butter and melt. Add the onion, mix and cook for 5 minutes. Add the stock, salt and pepper and put the steamer basket in the Instant Pot also.
2. Add the potatoes, cover the Instant Pot and cook for 5 minutes in the Manual setting. In a bowl, mix 3 tablespoons of butter with breadcrumbs and mix well. Relieve the pressure of the Instant Pot, remove the steam basket and transfer the potatoes to a pan.
3. Pour the cream and cheese into the instant pot and mix. Add the potatoes and mix gently.
4. Spread breadcrumbs, mix everywhere, place on a preheated grill and cook for 7 minutes. Let cool for a few minutes and serve.

- **Nutrition Info:** Calories: 340, Fat: 22, Fiber: 2, Carbohydrate: 32, Proteins: 11

29. Savory Chicken Nuggets With Parmesan Cheese

Servings: 4
Cooking Time: 25 Minutes
Ingredients:
- 1 lb chicken breasts, cubed
- Salt and black pepper to taste
- 2 tbsp olive oil
- 5 tbsp plain breadcrumbs
- 2 tbsp panko breadcrumbs
- 2 tbsp grated Parmesan cheese

Directions:
1. Preheat on Air Fry function to 380 F. Season the chicken with salt and pepper; set aside. In a bowl, mix the breadcrumbs with the Parmesan cheese.
2. Brush the chicken pieces with the olive oil, then dip into breadcrumb mixture, and transfer to the Air Fryer basket. Fit in the baking tray and lightly spray chicken with cooking spray. Cook for 10 minutes, flipping once halfway through until golden brown on the outside and no more pink on the inside. Serve warm.

30. Sausage Mushroom Caps(1)

Servings: 2
Cooking Time: 20 Minutes
Ingredients:
- ½ lb. Italian sausage
- 6 large Portobello mushroom caps
- ¼ cup grated Parmesan cheese.
- ¼ cup chopped onion
- 2 tbsp. blanched finely ground almond flour
- 1 tsp. minced fresh garlic

Directions:
1. Use a spoon to hollow out each mushroom cap, reserving scrapings.
2. In a medium skillet over medium heat, brown the sausage about 10 minutes or until fully cooked and no pink remains. Drain and then add reserved mushroom scrapings, onion, almond flour, Parmesan and garlic.
3. Gently fold ingredients together and continue cooking an additional minute, then remove from heat
4. Evenly spoon the mixture into mushroom caps and place the caps into a 6-inch round pan. Place pan into the air fryer basket
5. Adjust the temperature to 375 Degrees F and set the timer for 8 minutes. When finished cooking, the tops will be browned and bubbling. Serve warm.
- **Nutrition Info:** Calories: 404; Protein: 23g; Fiber: 5g; Fat: 28g; Carbs: 12g

31. Garlicky Roasted Chicken With Lemon

Servings:4
Cooking Time: 60 Minutes
Ingredients:
- 1 whole chicken (around 3.5 lb)
- 1 tbsp olive oil
- Salt and black pepper to taste
- 1 lemon, cut into quarters
- 5 garlic cloves

Directions:
1. Rub the chicken with olive oil and season with salt and pepper. Stuff the cavity with lemon and garlic. Place chicken, breast-side down on a baking tray. Tuck the legs and wings tips under.
2. Select Bake function, adjust the temperature to 360 F, and press Start. Bake for 30 minutes, turn breast-side up, and bake it for another 15 minutes. Let rest for 5-6 minutes then carve.

32. Sweet Pickle Chips With Buttermilk

Servings: 3
Cooking Time: 20 Minutes
Ingredients:
- 36 sweet pickle chips
- 1 cup buttermilk
- 3 tbsp smoked paprika
- 2 cups flour
- ¼ cup cornmeal
- Salt and black pepper to taste

Directions:
1. Preheat on Air Fryer function to 400 F. In a bowl, mix flour, paprika, pepper, salt, cornmeal, and powder. Place pickles in buttermilk and set aside for 5 minutes. Dip the pickles in the spice mixture and place them in the greased air fryer basket. Fit in the baking tray and cook for 10 minutes. Serve warm.

33. Risotto Bites

Servings: 4
Cooking Time: 10 Minutes
Ingredients:
- 1½ cups cooked risotto
- 3 tablespoons Parmesan cheese, grated
- ½ egg, beaten
- 1½ oz. mozzarella cheese, cubed
- 1/3 cup breadcrumbs

Directions:
1. In a bowl, add the risotto, Parmesan and egg and mix until well combined.
2. Make 20 equal-sized balls from the mixture.
3. Insert a mozzarella cube in the center of each ball.
4. With your fingers smooth the risotto mixture to cover the ball.
5. In a shallow dish, place the breadcrumbs.

6. Coat the balls with the breadcrumbs evenly.
7. Press "Power Button" of Air Fry Oven and turn the dial to select the "Air Fry" mode.
8. Press the Time button and again turn the dial to set the cooking time to 10 minutes.
9. Now push the Temp button and rotate the dial to set the temperature at 390 degrees F.
10. Press "Start/Pause" button to start.
11. When the unit beeps to show that it is preheated, open the lid.
12. Arrange the balls in "Air Fry Basket" and insert in the oven.
13. Serve warm.
- **Nutrition Info:** Calories 340 Total Fat 4.3 g Saturated Fat 2 g Cholesterol 29 mg Sodium 173 mg Total Carbs 62.4 g Fiber 1.3 g Sugar 0.7 g Protein 11.3 g

34. Roasted Vegetable And Kale Salad

Servings: 4
Cooking Time: 40 Minutes
Ingredients:
- 1 bunch kale, stems removed and chopped into ribbons
- 4 small or 2 large beets, peeled and cut roughly into 1-inch pieces
- 1/2 small butternut squash, peeled and cubed into 1-inch pieces
- 1 small red onion, sliced into 8 wedges
- 1 medium fennel bulb, sliced into 8 wedges
- 1 red pepper
- 3 tablespoons olive oil
- 1/2 cup coarsely chopped walnuts
- 3/4 teaspoon salt
- Pepper to taste
- 2 ounces goat cheese

Directions:
1. Cut the beets and pepper into one-inch pieces.
2. Remove the stems from the kale and chop into thin pieces.
3. Cut fennel and red onion into wedges.
4. Preheat the toaster oven to 425°F.
5. Toss together all vegetables, except kale, in a large bowl with oil, salt, and pepper.
6. Spread over a baking sheet and roast for 40 minutes turning halfway through.
7. At the 30-minute mark, remove tray from oven and sprinkle walnuts over and around vegetables.
8. Toss kale with dressing of choice and top with vegetables. Crumble goat cheese over salad and serve.
- **Nutrition Info:** Calories: 321, Sodium: 569 mg, Dietary Fiber: 5.5 g, Total Fat: 25.1 g, Total Carbs: 17.5 g, Protein: 11.1 g.

35. Crusted Brussels Sprouts With Sage

Servings:4

Cooking Time: 15 Minutes
Ingredients:
- 1 pound (454 g) Brussels sprouts, halved
- 1 cup bread crumbs
- 2 tablespoons grated Grana Padano cheese
- 1 tablespoon paprika
- 2 tablespoons canola oil
- 1 tablespoon chopped sage

Directions:
1. Line the air fryer basket with parchment paper. Set aside.
2. In a small bowl, thoroughly mix the bread crumbs, cheese, and paprika. In a large bowl, place the Brussels sprouts and drizzle the canola oil over the top. Sprinkle with the bread crumb mixture and toss to coat.
3. Transfer the Brussels sprouts to the prepared basket.
4. Put the air fryer basket on the baking pan and slide into Rack Position 2, select Roast, set temperature to 400ºF (205ºC), and set time to 15 minutes.
5. Stir the Brussels a few times during cooking.
6. When cooking is complete, the Brussels sprouts should be lightly browned and crisp. Transfer the Brussels sprouts to a plate and sprinkle the sage on top before serving.

36. Mom's Tarragon Chicken Breast Packets

Servings: 2
Cooking Time: 15 Minutes
Ingredients:
- 2 chicken breasts
- 1 tbsp butter
- Salt and black pepper to taste
- ¼ tsp dried tarragon

Directions:
1. Preheat on Bake function to 380 F. Place each chicken breast on a 12x12 inches foil wrap. Top the chicken with tarragon and butter; season with salt and pepper. Wrap the foil around the chicken breast in a loose way to create a flow of air. Cook the in your oven for 15 minutes. Carefully unwrap and serve.

37. Herbed Radish Sauté(1)

Servings: 4
Cooking Time: 20 Minutes
Ingredients:
- 2 bunches red radishes; halved
- 2 tbsp. parsley; chopped.
- 2 tbsp. balsamic vinegar
- 1 tbsp. olive oil
- Salt and black pepper to taste.

Directions:

1. Take a bowl and mix the radishes with the remaining ingredients except the parsley, toss and put them in your air fryer's basket.
2. Cook at 400°F for 15 minutes, divide between plates, sprinkle the parsley on top and serve as a side dish
- **Nutrition Info:** Calories: 180; Fat: 4g; Fiber: 2g; Carbs: 3g; Protein: 5g

38. Flavored Mashed Sweet Potatoes

Servings: 8
Cooking Time: 9 Minutes
Ingredients:
- 3 pounds sweet potatoes, peeled and chopped
- Salt and ground black pepper, to taste
- 2 garlic cloves
- ½ teaspoon dried parsley
- ½ teaspoon dried rosemary
- ¼ teaspoon dried sage
- ½ teaspoon dried thyme
- 1½ cups water
- ½ cup Parmesan cheese, grated
- 2 tablespoon butter
- ¼ cup milk

Directions:
1. Place the potatoes and garlic in the Instant Pot, add 1 ½ cups of water to the Instant Pot, cover and cook for 10 minutes in the manual setting.
2. Relieve the pressure, drain the water, transfer the potatoes and garlic to a bowl and mix them using a hand mixer.
3. Add butter, cheese, milk, salt, pepper, parsley, sage, rosemary and thyme and mix well. Divide between plates and serve.
- **Nutrition Info:** Calories: 240, Fat: 1, Fiber: 8.2, Carbohydrate: 34, Proteins: 4.5

39. Mustard Cheddar Twists

Servings:4
Cooking Time: 45 Minutes
Ingredients:
- 2 cups cauliflower florets, steamed
- 1 egg
- 3 ½ oz oats
- 1 red onion, diced
- 1 tsp mustard
- 5 oz cheddar cheese
- Salt and black pepper to taste

Directions:
1. Place the oats in a food processor and pulse until they resemble breadcrumbs. Place the steamed florets in a cheesecloth and squeeze out the excess liquid.
2. Transfer to a large bowl. Add in the rest of the ingredients. Mix well. Take a little bit of the mixture and twist it into a straw.

3. Place on a lined baking tray and repeat with the rest of the mixture. Select AirFry function, adjust the temperature to 360 F, and press Start. Cook for 10 minutes, turn over and cook for an additional 10 minutes.

40. Roasted Brussels Sprouts

Servings: 6
Cooking Time: 30 Minutes
Ingredients:
- 1-1/2 pounds Brussels sprouts, ends trimmed and yellow leaves removed
- 3 tablespoons olive oil
- 1 teaspoon salt
- 1/2 teaspoon black pepper

Directions:
1. Start by preheating toaster oven to 400°F.
2. Toss Brussels sprouts in a large bowl, drizzle with olive oil, sprinkle with salt and pepper, then toss.
3. Roast for 30 minutes.
- **Nutrition Info:** Calories: 109, Sodium: 416 mg, Dietary Fiber: 4.3 g, Total Fat: 7.4 g, Total Carbs: 10.4 g, Protein: 3.9 g.

41. French Fries

Servings: 4
Cooking Time: 10 Minutes
Ingredients:
- ¼ teaspoon baking soda Oil for frying
- Salt, to taste
- 8 medium potatoes, peeled, cut into medium matchsticks, and patted dry
- 1 cup water

Directions:
1. Put the water in the Instant Pot, add the salt and baking soda and mix. Place the potatoes in the steam basket and place them in the Instant Pot, cover and cook with manual adjustment for 3 minutes.
2. Release the pressure naturally, remove the chips from the Instant Pot and place them in a bowl. Heat a pan with enough oil over medium-high heat, add the potatoes, spread and cook until they are golden brown.
3. Transfer the potatoes to the paper towels to drain the excess fat and place them in a bowl. Salt, mix well and serve.
- **Nutrition Info:** Calories: 300, Fat: 10, Fiber: 3.7, Carbohydrate: 41, Proteins: 3.4

42. Avocado Fries

Servings: 4
Cooking Time: 20 Minutes
Ingredients:
- 1 oz. pork rinds, finely ground
- 2 medium avocados

Directions:

1. Cut each avocado in half. Remove the pit. Carefully remove the peel and then slice the flesh into ¼-inch-thick slices.
2. Place the pork rinds into a medium bowl and press each piece of avocado into the pork rinds to coat completely. Place the avocado pieces into the air fryer basket. Adjust the temperature to 350 Degrees F and set the timer for 5 minutes. Serve immediately
- **Nutrition Info:** Calories: 153; Protein: 4g; Fiber: 6g; Fat: 19g; Carbs: 9g

43. Cheesy Squash Casserole

Servings: 6
Cooking Time: 30 Minutes
Ingredients:
- 2 lbs yellow summer squash, cut into chunks
- 1/2 cup liquid egg substitute
- 3/4 cup cheddar cheese, shredded
- 1/4 cup mayonnaise
- 1/4 tsp salt

Directions:
1. Fit the oven with the rack in position
2. Add squash in a saucepan then pour enough water in a saucepan to cover the squash. Bring to boil.
3. Turn heat to medium and cook for 10 minutes or until tender. Drain well.
4. In a large mixing bowl, combine together squash, egg substitute, mayonnaise, 1/2 cup cheese, and salt.
5. Transfer squash mixture into a greased baking dish.
6. Set to bake at 375 F for 35 minutes. After 5 minutes place the baking dish in the preheated oven.
7. Sprinkle remaining cheese on top.
8. Serve and enjoy.
- **Nutrition Info:** Calories 130 Fat 8.2 g Carbohydrates 7.7 g Sugar 3.5 g Protein 8 g Cholesterol 18 mg

44. Parmesan Chicken Nuggets

Servings:4
Cooking Time: 25 Minutes
Ingredients:
- 1 lb chicken breast, cubed
- Salt and black pepper to taste
- 2 tbsp olive oil
- 5 tbsp plain breadcrumbs
- 2 tbsp panko breadcrumbs
- 2 tbsp grated Parmesan cheese

Directions:
1. Preheat on AirFry function to 380 F. Season the chicken with salt and pepper and drizzle with the olive oil. In a bowl, mix the crumbs with Parmesan cheese.

2. Coat the chicken pieces with the breadcrumb mixture and transfer them to the frying basket. Lightly grease chicken with cooking spray. Press Start. Cook the chicken for 10 minutes until golden brown on the outside and cooked on the inside. Serve warm.

45. Mango Cashew Nuts

Servings:2
Cooking Time: 25 Minutes
Ingredients:
- 1 cup Greek yogurt
- 2 tbsp mango powder
- ½ cup cashew nuts
- Salt and black pepper to taste
- 1 tsp coriander powder
- ½ tsp masala powder

Directions:
1. Preheat on Bake function to 360 F. In a bowl, mix all powders. Season with salt and pepper. Add cashews and toss to coat. Place in the oven and press Start. Cook for 15 minutes.

46. Homemade Tortilla Chips

Servings: 4
Cooking Time: 55 Minutes
Ingredients:
- 1 cup flour
- Salt and black pepper to taste
- 1 tbsp golden flaxseed meal
- 2 cups shredded Cheddar cheese

Directions:
1. Melt cheddar cheese in the microwave for 1 minute. Add flour, salt, flaxseed meal, and pepper. Mix well with a fork. On a board, place the dough and knead it with hands while warm until the ingredients are well combined. Divide the dough into 2 and with a rolling pin, roll them out flat into 2 rectangles. Use a pastry cutter to cut out triangle-shaped pieces.
2. Line them in one layer on the Air Fryer basket and spray with cooking spray. Fit in the baking tray and cook for 10 minutes on Air Fry function at 400 F. Serve with a cheese dip.

47. Zucchini Spaghetti

Servings: 4
Cooking Time: 20 Minutes
Ingredients:
- 1 lb. zucchinis, cut with a spiralizer
- 1 cup parmesan; grated
- ¼ cup parsley; chopped.
- ¼ cup olive oil
- 6 garlic cloves; minced
- ½ tsp. red pepper flakes

- Salt and black pepper to taste.

Directions:
1. In a pan that fits your air fryer, mix all the ingredients, toss, introduce in the fryer and cook at 370°F for 15 minutes
2. Divide between plates and serve as a side dish.
- **Nutrition Info:** Calories: 200; Fat: 6g; Fiber: 3g; Carbs: 4g; Protein: 5g

48. Beef Enchilada Dip

Servings: 8
Cooking Time: 10 Minutes
Ingredients:
- 2 lbs. ground beef
- ½ onion, chopped fine
- 2 cloves garlic, chopped fine
- 2 cups enchilada sauce
- 2 cups Monterrey Jack cheese, grated
- 2 tbsp. sour cream

Directions:
1. Place rack in position
2. Heat a large skillet over med-high heat. Add beef and cook until it starts to brown. Drain off fat.
3. Stir in onion and garlic and cook until tender, about 3 minutes. Stir in enchilada sauce and transfer mixture to a small casserole dish and top with cheese.
4. Set oven to convection bake on 325°F for 10 minutes. After 5 minutes, add casserole to the oven and bake 3-5 minutes until cheese is melted and mixture is heated through.
5. Serve warm topped with sour cream.
- **Nutrition Info:** Calories 414, Total Fat 22g, Saturated Fat 10g, Total Carbs 15g, Net Carbs 11g, Protein 39g, Sugar 8g, Fiber 4g, Sodium 1155mg, Potassium 635mg, Phosphorus 385mg

49. Mashed Turnips

Servings: 4
Cooking Time: 5 Minutes
Ingredients:
- ½ cup chicken stock
- 4 turnips, peeled and chopped
- ¼ cup sour cream
- Salt and ground black pepper, to taste
- 1 yellow onion, peeled and chopped

Directions:
1. In the Instant Pot, mix the turnips with the stock and onion. Stir, cover and cook in manual setting for 5 minutes.
2. Release the pressure naturally, drain the turnips and transfer to a bowl. Mix them using a food processor and add salt and pepper to taste and sour cream. Mix again and serve.

- **Nutrition Info:** Calories: 70, Fat: 1, Fiber: 4.6, Carbohydrate: 11.2, Proteins: 1.6

50. Balsamic Keto Vegetables

Servings: 3
Cooking Time: 20 Minutes
Ingredients:
- 1/2-pound cauliflower florets
- 1/2-pound button mushrooms, whole
- 1 cup pearl onions, whole
- Pink Himalayan salt and ground black pepper, to taste
- 1/4 teaspoon smoked paprika
- 1 teaspoon garlic powder
- 1/2 teaspoon dried thyme
- 1/2 teaspoon dried marjoram
- 3 tablespoons olive oil
- 2 tablespoons balsamic vinegar

Directions:
1. Toss all ingredients in a large mixing dish.
2. Roast in the preheated Air Fryer at 400 degrees F for 5 minutes. Shake the basket and cook for 7 minutes more.
3. Serve with some extra fresh herbs if desired.
- **Nutrition Info:** 170 Calories; 14g Fat; 7g Carbs; 2g Protein; 5g Sugars; 9g Fiber

51. Charred Green Beans With Sesame Seeds

Servings:4
Cooking Time: 8 Minutes
Ingredients:
- 1 tablespoon reduced-sodium soy sauce or tamari
- ½ tablespoon Sriracha sauce
- 4 teaspoons toasted sesame oil, divided
- 12 ounces (340 g) trimmed green beans
- ½ tablespoon toasted sesame seeds

Directions:
1. Whisk together the soy sauce, Sriracha sauce, and 1 teaspoon of sesame oil in a small bowl until smooth. Set aside.
2. Toss the green beans with the remaining sesame oil in a large bowl until evenly coated.
3. Place the green beans in the air fryer basket in a single layer.
4. Put the air fryer basket on the baking pan and slide into Rack Position 2, select Air Fry, set temperature to 375ºF (190ºC), and set time to 8 minutes.
5. Stir the green beans halfway through the cooking time.
6. When cooking is complete, the green beans should be lightly charred and tender. Remove from the oven to a platter. Pour the prepared sauce over the top of green beans and toss well. Serve sprinkled with the toasted sesame seeds.

52. Tasty Carrot Chips

Servings: 2
Cooking Time: 20 Minutes
Ingredients:
- 3 large carrots, washed and peeled
- Salt to taste

Directions:
1. Using a mandolin slicer, slice the carrots very thinly heightwise. Put the carrot strips in a bowl and season with salt. Grease the fryer basket lightly with cooking spray, and add the carrot strips. Fit in the baking tray and cook in the at 350 F for 10 minutes on Air Fry function, stirring once halfway through. Serve warm.

53. Lemon-garlic Kale Salad

Servings: 8
Cooking Time: 10 Minutes
Ingredients:
- 2 cups sliced almonds
- 1/3 cup lemon juice
- 1 teaspoon salt
- 1-1/2 cups olive oil
- 4 cloves crushed garlic
- 12 ounces kale, stems removed

Directions:
1. Set toaster oven to toast and toast almonds for about 5 minutes.
2. Combine lemon juice and salt in a small bowl, then add olive oil and garlic; mix well and set aside.
3. Slice kale into thin ribbons; place in a bowl and sprinkle with almonds.
4. Remove garlic from dressing, then add desired amount of dressing to kale and toss.
5. Add additional dressing if necessary, and serve.
- **Nutrition Info:** Calories: 487, Sodium: 312 mg, Dietary Fiber: 3.7 g, Total Fat: 49.8 g, Total Carbs: 10.2 g, Protein: 6.5 g.

54. Savory Curly Potatoes

Servings: 2
Cooking Time: 20 Minutes
Ingredients:
- 2 potatoes, spiralized
- 1 tbsp extra-virgin olive oil
- Salt and black pepper to taste
- 1 tsp paprika

Directions:
1. Preheat on Air Fry function to 350 F. Place the potatoes in a bowl and coat with oil. Transfer them to the cooking basket and fit in the baking tray. Cook for 15 minutes, shaking once. Sprinkle with salt, pepper, and paprika and to serve.

55. Roasted Tomatoes

Servings: 4
Cooking Time: 20 Minutes
Ingredients:
- 4 tomatoes; halved
- ½ cup parmesan; grated
- 1 tbsp. basil; chopped.
- ½ tsp. onion powder
- ½ tsp. oregano; dried
- ½ tsp. smoked paprika
- ½ tsp. garlic powder
- Cooking spray

Directions:
1. Take a bowl and mix all the ingredients except the cooking spray and the parmesan.
2. Arrange the tomatoes in your air fryer's pan, sprinkle the parmesan on top and grease with cooking spray
3. Cook at 370°F for 15 minutes, divide between plates and serve.
- **Nutrition Info:** Calories: 200; Fat: 7g; Fiber: 2g; Carbs: 4g; Protein: 6g

56. Butterbeans With Feta & Bacon

Servings:2
Cooking Time: 20 Minutes
Ingredients:
- 1 (14 oz) can butter beans
- 1 tbsp fresh chives, chopped
- ½ cup feta cheese, crumbled
- Black pepper to taste
- 1 tsp olive oil
- 2 oz bacon, sliced

Directions:
1. Preheat on AirFry function to 340 F. Blitz beans, oil, and pepper in a small blender. Arrange bacon slices on the frying basket.
2. Top with chives and place in the oven. Press Start and cook for 12 minutes. Add feta to the bean mixture and stir. Serve bacon with the dip.

57. Cheesy Sticks With Thai Sauce

Servings: 4
Cooking Time: 20 Minutes + Freezing Time
Ingredients:
- 12 mozzarella string cheese
- 2 cups breadcrumbs
- 3 eggs
- 1 cup sweet Thai sauce
- 4 tbsp skimmed milk

Directions:
1. Pour the crumbs in a bowl. Crack the eggs into another bowl and beat with the milk. One after the other, dip each cheese sticks in the egg mixture, in the crumbs, then egg mixture again and then in the crumbs back. Place the cheese sticks in a cookie sheet and freeze for 2 hours.

2. Preheat on Air Fry function to 380 F. Arrange the sticks in the frying basket without overcrowding. Fit in the baking tray and cook for 8 minutes, flipping them halfway through cooking until browned. Serve with the Thai sauce.

58. Pancetta & Hot Dogs Omelet

Servings: 2
Cooking Time: 10 Minutes
Ingredients:

- 4 eggs
- ¼ teaspoon dried parsley
- ¼ teaspoon dried rosemary
- 1 pancetta slice, chopped
- 2 hot dogs, chopped
- 2 small onions, chopped

Directions:

1. In a bowl, crack the eggs and beat well.
2. Add the remaining ingredients and gently, stir to combine.
3. Place the mixture into a baking pan.
4. Press "Power Button" of Air Fry Oven and turn the dial to select the "Air Fry" mode.
5. Press the Time button and again turn the dial to set the cooking time to 10 minutes.
6. Now push the Temp button and rotate the dial to set the temperature at 320 degrees F.
7. Press "Start/Pause" button to start.
8. When the unit beeps to show that it is preheated, open the lid.
9. Arrange pan over the "Wire Rack" and insert in the oven.
10. Cut into equal-sized wedges and serve hot.
- **Nutrition Info:** Calories 282 Total Fat 19.3 g Saturated Fat 6.5 g Cholesterol 351mg Sodium 632 mg Total Carbs 8.2 g Fiber 1.6 g Sugar 4.2 g Protein 18.9 g

59. Easy French Toast Casserole

Servings:6
Cooking Time: 12 Minutes
Ingredients:

- 3 large eggs, beaten
- 1 cup whole milk
- 1 tablespoon pure maple syrup
- 1 teaspoon vanilla extract
- ¼ teaspoon cinnamon
- ¼ teaspoon kosher salt
- 3 cups stale bread cubes
- 1 tablespoon unsalted butter, at room temperature
- In a medium bowl, whisk together the eggs, milk, maple syrup, vanilla extract, cinnamon and salt. Stir in the bread cubes to coat well.

Directions:

1. Grease the bottom of the baking pan with the butter. Spread the bread mixture into the pan in an even layer.
2. Slide the baking pan into Rack Position 2, select Roast, set temperature to 350ºF (180ºC) and set time to 12 minutes.
3. After about 10 minutes, remove the pan and check the casserole. The top should be browned and the middle of the casserole just set. If more time is needed, return the pan to the oven and continue cooking.
4. When cooking is complete, serve warm.

60. Easy Apple Pie Baked Oatmeal

Servings: 4
Cooking Time: 30 Minutes
Ingredients:

- 1 cup rolled oats
- 1/4 tsp nutmeg
- 2 tsp cinnamon
- 2 tbsp maple syrup
- 1/4 cup milk
- 1/2 cup raisins
- 1 banana, sliced
- 2 apples, diced
- 1 cup boiling water

Directions:

1. Fit the oven with the rack in position
2. Add oats and boiling water in a mixing bowl and let sit for 10 minutes.
3. After 10 minutes add remaining ingredients to the bowl and mix well.
4. Pour mixture into the greased baking dish.
5. Set to bake at 350 F for 35 minutes. After 5 minutes place the baking dish in the preheated oven.
6. Serve and enjoy.
- **Nutrition Info:** Calories 253 Fat 2.1 g Carbohydrates 58.8 g Sugar 32.8 g Protein 4.4 g Cholesterol 1 mg

61. Brioche Breakfast Pudding

Servings: 8
Cooking Time: 45 Minutes
Ingredients:

- 1 loaf brioche bread, cut in cubes
- ½ tbsp. coconut oil, soft
- 4 cups milk
- 1 can coconut milk
- 6 eggs
- ½ cup sugar
- 2 tsp vanilla
- ¼ tsp salt
- 1 cup coconut, shredded
- ½ cup chocolate chips

Directions:

1. Place rack in position 1 of the oven. Grease an 8x11-inch baking pan with coconut oil.
2. Add the bread cubes to the pan, pressing lightly to settle.
3. In a large bowl, whisk together milk, coconut milk, eggs, sugar, vanilla, and salt until combined.
4. Stir in coconut and chocolate chips. Pour evenly over bread. Cover with plastic wrap and refrigerate 2 hours or overnight.

5. Set oven to bake on 350°F for 50 minutes. After 5 minutes, add the pudding to the oven and bake 40-45 minutes, or until top is beginning to brown and it passes the toothpick test.
6. Remove to wire rack and let cool 5-10 minutes before serving.
- **Nutrition Info:** Calories 476, Total Fat 24g, Saturated Fat 15g, Total Carbs 51g, Net Carbs 48g, Protein 14g, Sugar 30g, Fiber 3g, Sodium 398mg, Potassium 443mg, Phosphorus 288mg

62. Grilled Cheese Sandwich

Servings: 1 Person
Cooking Time: 12 Minutes
Ingredients:
- 2 slices of bread
- 2 pieces of bacon
- ½ tsp of olive oil side
- Tomatoes
- Jack cheese
- Peach preserves

Directions:
1. If you have left over bacon from air fried bacon recipe you can get two pieces. However, if you do not have any leftover bacon you can get two pieces and fry them at 200 degree Celsius.
2. Place olive oil on the side of the bread slices. Layer the rest of the ingredients on the non-oiled side following the following steps, peach preserves, tomatoes, jack cheese and cooked bacon.
3. Press down the bread to allow it to cook a little bit and peach side down too to allow the bread and the peel to spread evenly.
4. Place the sandwich in an air fryer and cook it for 12 minutes
5. at 393 degrees Fahrenheit.
6. Serve once you are done.
- **Nutrition Info:** Calories 282 Fats 18g, Carbs 18g, Proteins 12g, Sodium: 830 Mg, Potassium: 250mg

63. Mushroom Sausage Breakfast Bake

Servings: 6
Cooking Time: 30 Minutes
Ingredients:
- 12 eggs
- 2 cups spinach, chopped
- 1 tbsp garlic, minced
- 8 oz mushrooms, sliced
- 1 red bell pepper, diced
- 1 small onion, diced
- 2 tbsp olive oil
- 7 oz sausage links, diced
- Pepper
- Salt

Directions:
1. Fit the oven with the rack in position
2. Spray 9*13-inch baking pan with cooking spray and set aside.
3. Heat oil in a pan over medium-high heat.
4. Add onion and bell pepper and sauté for 2-3 minutes.
5. Add garlic and mushrooms and sauté for 2 minutes.
6. Add sausage and spinach and cook until heated through.
7. Spread pan mixture into the greased baking pan.
8. In a bowl, whisk eggs with pepper and salt.
9. Pour egg mixture over sausage mixture.
10. Set to bake at 350 F for 35 minutes. After 5 minutes place the baking pan in the preheated oven.
11. Serve and enjoy.
- **Nutrition Info:** Calories 293 Fat 23 g Carbohydrates 6 g Sugar 3.2 g Protein 16.9 g Cholesterol 348 mg

64. Caprese Sourdough Sandwich

Servings:2
Cooking Time: 25 Minutes
Ingredients:
- 4 sourdough bread slices
- 2 tbsp mayonnaise
- 2 slices ham
- 2 lettuce leaves
- 1 tomato, sliced
- 2 mozzarella cheese slices
- Salt and black pepper to taste

Directions:
1. On a clean board, lay the sourdough slices and spread with mayonnaise. Top 2 of the slices with ham, lettuce, tomato and mozzarella. Season with salt and pepper. Top with the remaining two slices to form two sandwiches. Spray with oil and transfer to the frying basket. Cook in the preheated oven for 14 minutes at 340 F on Bake function.

65. Moist Orange Bread Loaf

Servings: 10
Cooking Time: 50 Minutes
Ingredients:
- 4 eggs
- 4 oz butter, softened
- 1 cup of orange juice
- 1 orange zest, grated
- 1 cup of sugar
- 2 tsp baking powder
- 2 cups all-purpose flour
- 1 tsp vanilla

Directions:
1. Fit the oven with the rack in position

2. In a large bowl, whisk eggs and sugar until creamy.
3. Whisk in vanilla, butter, orange juice, and orange zest.
4. Add flour and baking powder and mix until combined.
5. Pour batter into the greased 9*5-inch loaf pan.
6. Set to bake at 350 F for 55 minutes, after 5 minutes, place the loaf pan in the oven.
7. Slice and serve.
- **Nutrition Info:** Calories 286 Fat 11.3 g Carbohydrates 42.5 g Sugar 22.4 g Protein 5.1 gCholesterol 90 mg

66. Mediterranean Spinach Frittata

Servings: 6
Cooking Time: 20 Minutes
Ingredients:
- 6 eggs
- 1/2 cup frozen spinach, drained the excess liquid
- 1/4 cup feta cheese, crumbled
- 1/4 cup olives, chopped
- 1/4 cup kalamata olives, chopped
- 1/2 cup tomatoes, diced
- 1/2 tsp garlic powder
- 1 tsp oregano
- 1/4 cup milk
- 1/2 tsp pepper
- 1/4 tsp salt

Directions:
1. Fit the oven with the rack in position
2. Spray 9-inch pie pan with cooking spray and set aside.
3. In a bowl, whisk eggs with oregano, garlic powder, milk, pepper, and salt until well combined.
4. Add olives, feta cheese, tomatoes, and spinach and mix well.
5. Pour egg mixture into the prepared pie pan.
6. Set to bake at 400 F for 25 minutes. After 5 minutes place the pie pan in the preheated oven.
7. Serve and enjoy.
- **Nutrition Info:** Calories 103 Fat 7.2 g Carbohydrates 2.9 g Sugar 1.5 g Protein 7.2 g Cholesterol 170 mg

67. Cinnamon-orange Toast

Servings: 6
Cooking Time: 15 Minutes
Ingredients:
- 12 slices bread
- ½ cup sugar
- 1 stick butter
- 1½ tbsp vanilla extract
- 1½ tbsp cinnamon
- 2 oranges, zested

Directions:
1. Mix butter, sugar, and vanilla extract and microwave for 30 seconds until everything melts. Add in orange zest. Pour the mixture over bread slices. Lay the bread slices in your Air Fryer pan and cook for 5 minutes at 400 F on Toast function. Serve with berry sauce.

68. Veggie Frittata

Servings:4
Cooking Time: 12 Minutes
Ingredients:
- ½ cup chopped red bell pepper
- $1/3$ cup grated carrot
- $1/3$ cup minced onion
- 1 teaspoon olive oil
- 1 egg
- 6 egg whites
- $1/3$ cup 2% milk
- 1 tablespoon shredded Parmesan cheese

Directions:
1. Mix together the red bell pepper, carrot, onion, and olive oil in the baking pan and stir to combine.
2. Slide the baking pan into Rack Position 1, select Convection Bake, set temperature to 350ºF (180ºC) and set time to 12 minutes.
3. After 3 minutes, remove the pan from the oven. Stir the vegetables. Return the pan to the oven and continue cooking.
4. Meantime, whisk together the egg, egg whites, and milk in a medium bowl until creamy.
5. After 3 minutes, remove the pan from the oven. Pour the egg mixture over the top and scatter with the Parmesan cheese. Return the pan to the oven and continue cooking for additional 6 minutes.
6. When cooking is complete, the eggs will be set and the top will be golden around the edges.
7. Allow the frittata to cool for 5 minutes before slicing and serving.

69. Yogurt & Cream Cheese Zucchini Cakes

Servings: 4
Cooking Time: 20 Minutes
Ingredients:
- 1 ½ cups flour
- 1 tsp cinnamon
- 3 eggs
- 2 tsp baking powder
- 2 tbsp sugar
- 1 cup milk
- 2 tbsp butter, melted
- 1 tbsp yogurt
- ½ cup shredded zucchini

- 2 tbsp cream cheese

Directions:
1. In a bowl, whisk the eggs along with the sugar, salt, cinnamon, cream cheese, flour, and baking powder. In another bowl, combine all of the liquid ingredients. Gently combine the dry and liquid mixtures. Stir in zucchini.
2. Line muffin tins with baking paper, and pour the batter inside them. Arrange on the Air Fryer tray and cook for 15-18 minutes on Bake function at 380 F. Serve chilled.

70. Apple-cinnamon Empanadas

Servings: 2-4
Cooking Time: 30 Minutes
Ingredients:
- 2-3 baking apples, peeled & diced
- 2 tsp.s of cinnamon
- 1/4 cup white sugar
- 1 tablespoon brown sugar
- 1 tablespoon of water
- 1/2 tablespoon cornstarch
- ¼ tsp. of vanilla extract
- 2 tablespoons of margarine or margarine
- 4 pre-made empanada dough shells (Goya)

Directions:
1. In a bowl, add together white sugar, brown sugar, cornstarch and cinnamon; set aside. Put the diced apples in a pot and place on a stovetop.
2. Add the combined dry ingredients to the apples, then add the water, vanilla extract, and margarine; stirring well to mix.
3. Cover pot and cook on high heat. Once it starts boiling, lower heat and simmer, until the apples are soft. Remove from the heat and cool.
4. Lay the empanada shells on a clean counter. Ladle the apple mixture into each of the shells, being careful to prevent spillage over the edges. Fold shells to fully cover apple mixture, seal edges with water, pressing down to secure with a fork.
5. Cover the air fryer basket with tin foil but leave the edges uncovered so that air can circulate through the basket. Place the empanadas shells in the foil lined air fryer basket, set temperature at 350°F and timer for 15 minutes.
6. Halfway through, slide the frying basket out and flip the empanadas using a spatula. Remove when golden, and serve directly from the basket onto plates.
- **Nutrition Info:** Calories 113 Fat 8.2 g Carbohydrates 0.3 g Sugar 0.2 g Protein 5.4 g Cholesterol 18 mg

71. Air Fried Philly Cheesesteaks

Servings:2
Cooking Time: 20 Minutes
Ingredients:
- 12 ounces (340 g) boneless rib-eye steak, sliced thinly
- ½ teaspoon Worcestershire sauce
- ½ teaspoon soy sauce
- Kosher salt and ground black pepper, to taste
- ½ green bell pepper, stemmed, deseeded, and thinly sliced
- ½ small onion, halved and thinly sliced
- 1 tablespoon vegetable oil
- 2 soft hoagie rolls, split three-fourths of the way through
- 1 tablespoon butter, softened
- 2 slices provolone cheese, halved

Directions:
1. Combine the steak, Worcestershire sauce, soy sauce, salt, and ground black pepper in a large bowl. Toss to coat well. Set aside.
2. Combine the bell pepper, onion, salt, ground black pepper, and vegetable oil in a separate bowl. Toss to coat the vegetables well.
3. Place the steak and vegetables in the air fryer basket.
4. Put the air fryer basket on the baking pan and slide into Rack Position 2, select Air Fry, set temperature to 400ºF (205ºC) and set time to 15 minutes.
5. When cooked, the steak will be browned and vegetables will be tender. Transfer them onto a plate. Set aside.
6. Brush the hoagie rolls with butter and place in the basket.
7. Select Toast and set time to 3 minutes. Return to the oven. When done, the rolls should be lightly browned.
8. Transfer the rolls to a clean work surface and divide the steak and vegetable mix between the rolls. Spread with cheese. Transfer the stuffed rolls to the basket.
9. Select Air Fry and set time to 2 minutes. Return to the oven. When done, the cheese should be melted.
10. Serve immediately.

72. Fluffy Frittata With Bell Pepper

Servings:x
Cooking Time:x
Ingredients:
- 8 eggs
- 2 Tbsp whole milk
- 1 Tbsp butter
- Coarse salt, freshly ground pepper, to taste
- ½ zucchini diced
- 1 bell Pepper seeded and diced

Directions:
1. Preheat oven to 400°F.
2. Heat oven over medium heat. Add butter.
3. In a bowl, add remaining ingredients. Pour mixture into oven.
4. When eggs are half set and edges begin to pull away, place frittata in
5. the oven and bake for about 10 minutes, or until center is no longer jiggly.
6. Cut into wedges or slide out onto serving plate.

73. Meat Lover Omelet With Mozzarella

Servings:2
Cooking Time: 20 Minutes
Ingredients:
- 1 beef sausage, chopped
- 4 slices prosciutto, chopped
- 3 oz salami, chopped
- 1 cup grated mozzarella cheese
- 4 eggs
- 1 tbsp chopped onion
- 1 tbsp ketchup

Directions:
1. Preheat on Bake function to 350 F. Whisk the eggs with ketchup in a bowl. Stir in the onion. Brown the sausage in a greased pan over medium heat for 2 minutes.
2. Combine the egg mixture, mozzarella cheese, salami, and prosciutto. Pour the egg mixture over the sausage and give it a stir. Press Start and cook in the for 15 minutes.

74. Bacon Bread Egg Casserole

Servings: 4
Cooking Time: 20 Minutes
Ingredients:
- 6 eggs
- 1 cup cheddar cheese, shredded
- 1/2 tsp garlic, minced
- 3 tbsp milk
- 2 tbsp green onion, chopped
- 1/3 bell pepper, diced
- 2 bread slices, cubed
- 5 bacon slices, diced
- Pepper
- Salt

Directions:
1. Fit the oven with the rack in position
2. Add all ingredients into the large bowl and stir until well combined.
3. Pour into the greased baking dish.
4. Set to bake at 350 F for 25 minutes. After 5 minutes place the baking dish in the preheated oven.
5. Serve and enjoy.
- **Nutrition Info:** Calories 231 Fat 26.3 g Carbohydrates 5.2 g Sugar 1.9 g Protein 25 g Cholesterol 302 mg

75. Avocado And Zucchini Mix

Servings: 4
Cooking Time: 15 Minutes
Ingredients:
- 2 avocados, peeled, pitted and roughly cubed
- 2 zucchinis, roughly cubed
- 1 tablespoon olive oil
- 2 spring onions, chopped
- 8 eggs, whisked
- 1 teaspoon sweet paprika
- A pinch of salt and black pepper
- 1 tablespoon dill, chopped

Directions:
1. Heat up the air fryer with the oil at 350 degrees F, add the zucchinis and the spring onions and cook for 2 minutes.
2. Add the avocados and the other ingredients, cook the mix for 13 minutes more, divide into bowls and serve.
- **Nutrition Info:** calories 232, fat 12, fiber 2, carbs 10, protein 5

76. Latkes

Servings: 5
Cooking Time: 7 Minutes
Ingredients:
- 1 large onion
- 5 large potatoes peeled
- 4 large eggs
- ¼ cup potato starch
- 2 tsp kosher salt
- ½ tsp baking powder
- Olive oil

Directions:
1. Scrub your potatoes well and place them in a food processor. Besides, place the shredded potatoes in a bowl of cool water and set it aside.
2. Rinse the food in the processor and grate the onions. Place your grated onions in a paper towel and squeeze out the liquid.
3. In a medium sized bowl whisk your eggs and add matzo, pepper, 1 tsp potato starch, baking powder and grated onion. Drain the water from the potatoes and save the starch that remains in your bowl.
4. Scoop the starch from the potato bowl and add to the latke mixture. Form latkes from the mixture in flat circles and dip into dry potato starch. Add oil and place them in an air fryer
5. Air fry your latkes at 360-degree Fahrenheit for 8 minutes
6. and turn in the middle once it indicates turn food.
7. Serve while hot.
- **Nutrition Info:** Calories 68 Fat 4g, Carbohydrates 6g, Protein 2g.

77. Simply Bacon

Servings: 1 Person
Cooking Time: 10 Minutes
Ingredients:
- 4 pieces of bacon

Directions:
1. Place the bacon strips on the instant vortex air fryer.
2. Cook for 10 minutes
3. at 200 degrees Celsius.
4. Check when it browns and shows to be ready. Serve.
- **Nutrition Info:** Calories 165, Fat 13g, Proteins 12 g, Carbs 0g

78. Cheesy Spring Chicken Wraps

Servings:12
Cooking Time: 5 Minutes
Ingredients:
- 2 large-sized chicken breasts, cooked and shredded
- 2 spring onions, chopped
- 10 ounces (284 g) Ricotta cheese
- 1 tablespoon rice vinegar
- 1 tablespoon molasses
- 1 teaspoon grated fresh ginger
- ¼ cup soy sauce
- $^1/_3$ teaspoon sea salt
- ¼ teaspoon ground black pepper, or more to taste
- 48 wonton wrappers
- Cooking spray

Directions:
1. Spritz the air fryer basket with cooking spray.
2. Combine all the ingredients, except for the wrappers in a large bowl. Toss to mix well.
3. Unfold the wrappers on a clean work surface, then divide and spoon the mixture in the middle of the wrappers.
4. Dab a little water on the edges of the wrappers, then fold the edge close to you over the filling. Tuck the edge under the filling and roll up to seal.
5. Arrange the wraps in the pan.
6. Put the air fryer basket on the baking pan and slide into Rack Position 2, select Air Fry, set temperature to 375ºF (190ºC) and set time to 5 minutes.
7. Flip the wraps halfway through the cooking time.
8. When cooking is complete, the wraps should be lightly browned.
9. Serve immediately.

79. Prosciutto & Mozzarella Crostini

Servings: 1
Cooking Time: 7 Minutes
Ingredients:
- ½ cup finely chopped tomatoes
- 3 oz chopped mozzarella
- 3 prosciutto slices, chopped
- 1 tbsp olive oil
- 1 tsp dried basil
- 6 small slices of French bread

Directions:
1. Preheat on Toast function to 350 F. Place the bread slices in the toaster oven and toast for 5 minutes. Top the bread with tomatoes, prosciutto and mozzarella. Sprinkle the basil over the mozzarella. Drizzle with olive oil. Return to oven and cook for 1 more minute, enough to become melty and warm.

80. Ham And Cheese Toast

Servings: 1
Cooking Time: 6 Minutes
Ingredients:
- 1 slice bread
- 1 teaspoon butter, at room temperature
- 1 egg
- Salt and freshly ground black pepper, to taste
- 2 teaspoons diced ham
- 1 tablespoon grated Cheddar cheese

Directions:
1. On a clean work surface, use a 2½-inch biscuit cutter to make a hole in the center of the bread slice with about ½-inch of bread remaining.
2. Spread the butter on both sides of the bread slice. Crack the egg into the hole and season with salt and pepper to taste. Transfer the bread to the air fryer basket.
3. Put the air fryer basket on the baking pan and slide into Rack Position 2, select Air Fry, set temperature to 325ºF (163ºC), and set time to 6 minutes.
4. After 5 minutes, remove the pan from the oven. Scatter the cheese and diced ham on top and continue cooking for an additional 1 minute.
5. When cooking is complete, the egg should be set and the cheese should be melted. Remove the toast from the oven to a plate and let cool for 5 minutes before serving.

81. Sweet Pineapple Oatmeal

Servings: 6
Cooking Time: 45 Minutes
Ingredients:
- 2 cups old-fashioned oats
- 1/2 cup coconut flakes
- 1 cup pineapple, crushed
- 2 eggs, lightly beaten
- 1/3 cup yogurt
- 1/3 cup butter, melted

- 1/2 tsp baking powder
- 1/3 cup brown sugar
- 1/2 tsp vanilla
- 2/3 cup milk
- 1/2 tsp salt

Directions:
1. Fit the oven with the rack in position
2. In a mixing bowl, mix together oats, baking powder, brown sugar, and salt.
3. In a separate bowl, beat eggs with vanilla, milk, yogurt, and butter.
4. Add egg mixture into the oat mixture and stir to combine.
5. Add coconut and pineapple and stir to combine.
6. Pour oat mixture into the greased 8-inch baking dish.
7. Set to bake at 350 F for 50 minutes, after 5 minutes, place the baking dish in the oven.
8. Serve and enjoy.
- **Nutrition Info:** Calories 304 Fat 16.4 g Carbohydrates 33.2 g Sugar 13.6 g Protein 7.5 g Cholesterol 85 mg

82. Breakfast Tater Tot Casserole

Servings:4
Cooking Time: 17 To 18 Minutes
Ingredients:
- 4 eggs
- 1 cup milk
- Salt and pepper, to taste
- 12 ounces (340 g) ground chicken sausage
- 1 pound (454 g) frozen tater tots, thawed
- ¾ cup grated Cheddar cheese
- Cooking spray

Directions:
1. Whisk together the eggs and milk in a medium bowl. Season with salt and pepper to taste and stir until mixed. Set aside.
2. Place a skillet over medium-high heat and spritz with cooking spray. Place the ground sausage in the skillet and break it into smaller pieces with a spatula or spoon. Cook for 3 to 4 minutes until the sausage starts to brown, stirring occasionally. Remove from heat and set aside.
3. Coat the baking pan with cooking spray. Arrange the tater tots in the baking pan.
4. Slide the baking pan into Rack Position 1, select Convection Bake, set temperature to 400ºF (205ºC) and set time to 14 minutes.
5. After 6 minutes, remove the pan from the oven. Stir the tater tots and add the egg mixture and cooked sausage. Return the pan to the oven and continue cooking.
6. After 6 minutes, remove the pan from the oven. Scatter the cheese on top of the tater tots. Return the pan to the oven and continue to cook for another 2 minutes.

7. When done, the cheese should be bubbly and melted.
8. Let the mixture cool for 5 minutes and serve warm.

83. Zucchini Breakfast Bread

Servings: 10
Cooking Time: 50 Minutes
Ingredients:
- 2 eggs
- 1 1/2 cups zucchini, grated
- 1 tsp vanilla extract
- 1/4 cup yogurt
- 1/2 tsp baking powder
- 1 1/2 cups whole wheat flour
- 1/2 cup applesauce
- 1/4 cup coconut sugar
- 1 tsp ground cinnamon
- 1/2 tsp baking soda
- 1/2 cup apple, grated
- 1/4 tsp sea salt

Directions:
1. Fit the oven with the rack in position
2. In a bowl, mix all dry ingredients.
3. In another bowl, whisk eggs, coconut sugar, vanilla, yogurt, and applesauce.
4. Add dry ingredients mixture into the wet mixture and stir until well combined.
5. Add apples and zucchini and stir well.
6. Pour batter into the 9*5-inch greased loaf pan.
7. Set to bake at 350 F for 55 minutes, after 5 minutes, place the loaf pan in the oven.
8. Slice and serve.
- **Nutrition Info:** Calories 103 Fat 1.2 g Carbohydrates 19.1 g Sugar 3.3 g Protein 3.7 g Cholesterol 33 mg

84. Baked Apple Breakfast Oats

Servings: 1
Cooking Time: 15 Minutes
Ingredients:
- 1/3 cup vanilla Greek yogurt
- 1/3 cup rolled oats
- 1 apple
- 1 tablespoon peanut butter

Directions:
1. Preheat toaster oven to 400°F and set it on the warm setting.
2. Cut apples into chunks approximately 1/2-inch-thick.
3. Place apples in an oven-safe dish with some space between each chunk and sprinkle with cinnamon.
4. Bake in the oven for 12 minutes.
5. Combine yogurt and oats in a bowl.
6. Remove the apples from the oven and combine with the yogurt.

7. Top with peanut butter for a delicious and high-protein breakfast.
- **Nutrition Info:** Calories: 350, Sodium: 134 mg, Dietary Fiber: 8.1 g, Total Fat: 11.2 g, Total Carbs: 52.5 g, Protein: 12.7 g.

85. Classic Cheddar Cheese Omelet

Servings: 1
Cooking Time: 15 Minutes
Ingredients:
- 2 eggs, beaten
- Black pepper to taste
- 1 cup cheddar cheese, shredded
- 1 whole onion, chopped
- 2 tbsp soy sauce

Directions:
1. Preheat on Air Fry function to 340 F. In a bowl, mix the eggs with soy sauce, salt, and pepper. Stir in the onion and cheddar cheese.
2. Pour the egg mixture in a greased baking pan and cook for 10-12 minutes. Serve and enjoy!

86. Balsamic Chicken With Spinach & Kale

Servings:1
Cooking Time: 20 Minutes
Ingredients:
- ½ cup baby spinach
- ½ cup romaine lettuce, shredded
- 3 large kale leaves, chopped
- 1 chicken breast, cut into cubes
- 2 tbsp olive oil
- 1 tsp balsamic vinegar
- 1 garlic clove, minced
- Salt and black pepper to taste

Directions:
1. Place the chicken, some olive oil, garlic, salt, and pepper in a bowl; toss to combine. Put on a lined baking dish and cook in the for 14 minutes at 390F on Bake function.
2. Meanwhile, place the greens in a large bowl. Add the remaining olive oil and balsamic vinegar. Season with salt and pepper and toss to combine. Top with the sliced chicken and serve.

87. Banana And Oat Bread Pudding

Servings:4
Cooking Time: 16 Minutes
Ingredients:
- 2 medium ripe bananas, mashed
- ½ cup low-fat milk
- 2 tablespoons maple syrup
- 2 tablespoons peanut butter
- 1 teaspoon vanilla extract
- 1 teaspoon ground cinnamon

- 2 slices whole-grain bread, cut into bite-sized cubes
- ¼ cup quick oats
- Cooking spray

Directions:
1. Spritz the baking pan lightly with cooking spray.
2. Mix the bananas, milk, maple syrup, peanut butter, vanilla, and cinnamon in a large mixing bowl and stir until well incorporated.
3. Add the bread cubes to the banana mixture and stir until thoroughly coated. Fold in the oats and stir to combine.
4. Transfer the mixture to the baking pan. Wrap the baking pan in aluminum foil.
5. Slide the baking pan into Rack Position 2, select Air Fry, set temperature to 350ºF (180ºC) and set time to 16 minutes.
6. After 10 minutes, remove the pan from the oven. Remove the foil. Return the pan to the oven and continue to cook for another 6 minutes.
7. When done, the pudding should be set.
8. Let the pudding cool for 5 minutes before serving.

88. Tomato Oatmeal

Servings: 4
Cooking Time: 20 Minutes
Ingredients:
- 1 cup tomatoes, cubed
- 1 cup old fashioned oats
- 2 cups almond milk
- A drizzle of avocado oil
- A pinch of salt and black pepper
- 1 teaspoon cilantro, chopped
- 1 teaspoon basil, chopped
- 2 spring onions, chopped

Directions:
1. In your air fryer, combine the tomatoes with the oats and the other ingredients, toss and cook at 360 degrees F for 20 minutes.
2. Divide the oatmeal into bowls and serve for breakfast.
- **Nutrition Info:** calories 140, fat 2, fiber 3, carbs 8, protein 4

89. Zucchini And Carrot Pudding

Servings: 4
Cooking Time: 15 Minutes
Ingredients:
- 1 cup carrots, shredded
- 1 cup zucchinis, grated
- 1 cup heavy cream
- 1 cup wild rice
- 2 cups coconut milk
- 1 teaspoon cardamom, ground
- 2 teaspoons sugar
- Cooking spray

Directions:

1. Spray your air fryer with cooking spray, add the carrots, zucchinis and the other ingredients, toss, cover and cook at 365 degrees F for 15 minutes.
2. Divide the pudding into bowls and serve for breakfast.
- **Nutrition Info:** calories 172, fat 7, fiber 4, carbs 14, protein 5

90. Avocado Cauliflower Toast

Servings: 2
Cooking Time: 30 Minutes
Ingredients:

- 1: 12-oz.steamer bag cauliflower
- ½ cup shredded mozzarella cheese
- 1 large egg.
- 1 ripe medium avocado
- ½ tsp. garlic powder.
- ¼ tsp. ground black pepper

Directions:

1. Cook cauliflower according to package instructions. Remove from bag and place into cheesecloth or clean towel to remove excess moisture.
2. Place cauliflower into a large bowl and mix in egg and mozzarella. Cut a piece of parchment to fit your air fryer basket
3. Separate the cauliflower mixture into two and place it on the parchment in two mounds. Press out the cauliflower mounds into a ¼-inch-thick rectangle. Place the parchment into the air fryer basket.
4. Adjust the temperature to 400 Degrees F and set the timer for 8 minutes
5. Flip the cauliflower halfway through the cooking time
6. When the timer beeps, remove the parchment and allow the cauliflower to cool 5 minutes.
7. Cut open the avocado and remove the pit. Scoop out the inside, place it in a medium bowl and mash it with garlic powder and pepper. Spread onto the cauliflower.
- **Nutrition Info:** Calories: 278; Protein: 14.1g; Fiber: 8.2g; Fat: 15.6g; Carbs: 15.9g

91. Ham Shirred Eggs With Parmesan

Servings:2
Cooking Time: 20 Minutes
Ingredients:

- 4 eggs
- 2 tbsp heavy cream
- 4 ham slices
- 3 tbsp Parmesan cheese, shredded
- ¼ tsp paprika
- Salt and black pepper to taste
- 2 tsp chives, chopped

Directions:

1. Preheat on AirFry function to 320 F. Arrange the ham slices on the bottom of a greased pan to cover it completely. Whisk 1 egg along with the heavy cream, salt, and pepper in a bowl.
2. Pour the mixture over the ham slices. Crack the other eggs on top. Sprinkle with Parmesan cheese and press Start. Cook for 14 minutes. Sprinkle with paprika and chives and serve.

92. Turkey Sliders With Chive Mayo

Servings:6
Cooking Time: 15 Minutes
Ingredients:

- 12 burger buns
- Cooking spray
- Turkey Sliders:
- ¾ pound (340 g) turkey, minced
- 1 tablespoon oyster sauce
- ¼ cup pickled jalapeno, chopped
- 2 tablespoons chopped scallions
- 1 tablespoon chopped fresh cilantro
- 1 to 2 cloves garlic, minced
- Sea salt and ground black pepper, to taste
- Chive Mayo:
- 1 tablespoon chives
- 1 cup mayonnaise
- Zest of 1 lime
- 1 teaspoon salt

Directions:

1. Spritz the air fryer basket with cooking spray.
2. Combine the ingredients for the turkey sliders in a large bowl. Stir to mix well. Shape the mixture into 6 balls, then bash the balls into patties.
3. Arrange the patties in the pan and spritz with cooking spray.
4. Put the air fryer basket on the baking pan and slide into Rack Position 2, select Air Fry, set temperature to 365ºF (185ºC) and set time to 15 minutes.
5. Flip the patties halfway through the cooking time.
6. Meanwhile, combine the ingredients for the chive mayo in a small bowl. Stir to mix well.
7. When cooked, the patties will be well browned.
8. Smear the patties with chive mayo, then assemble the patties between two buns to make the sliders. Serve immediately.

93. Crispy Tilapia Tacos

Servings:4
Cooking Time: 5 Minutes
Ingredients:

- 2 tablespoons milk
- $^1/_3$ cup mayonnaise

- ¼ teaspoon garlic powder
- 1 teaspoon chili powder
- 1½ cups panko bread crumbs
- ½ teaspoon salt
- 4 teaspoons canola oil
- 1 pound (454 g) skinless tilapia fillets, cut into 3-inch-long and 1-inch-wide strips
- 4 small flour tortillas
- Lemon wedges, for topping
- Cooking spray

Directions:
1. Spritz the air fryer basket with cooking spray.
2. Combine the milk, mayo, garlic powder, and chili powder in a bowl. Stir to mix well. Combine the panko with salt and canola oil in a separate bowl. Stir to mix well.
3. Dredge the tilapia strips in the milk mixture first, then dunk the strips in the panko mixture to coat well. Shake the excess off.
4. Arrange the tilapia strips in the pan.
5. Put the air fryer basket on the baking pan and slide into Rack Position 2, select Air Fry, set temperature to 400ºF (205ºC) and set time to 5 minutes.
6. Flip the strips halfway through the cooking time.
7. When cooking is complete, the strips will be opaque on all sides and the panko will be golden brown.
8. Unfold the tortillas on a large plate, then divide the tilapia strips over the tortillas. Squeeze the lemon wedges on top before serving.

94. Buttery Chocolate Toast

Servings: 1
Cooking Time: 5 Minutes
Ingredients:
- Whole wheat bread slices
- Coconut oil
- Pure maple syrup
- Cacao powder

Directions:
1. Toast the bread in toaster oven.
2. Spread coconut oil over the toast.
3. Drizzle maple syrup in lines over the toast.
4. Sprinkle cacao powder and serve.
- **Nutrition Info:** Calories: 101, Sodium: 133 mg, Dietary Fiber: 2.4 g, Total Fat: 3.5 g, Total Carbs: 14.8 g, Protein: 4.0 g.

95. Quick Paprika Eggs

Servings: 4
Cooking Time: 10 Minutes
Ingredients:
- 4 large eggs
- 1 tsp paprika
- Salt and pepper to taste

- ¼ cup cottage cheese, crumbled

Directions:
1. Preheat your fryer to 350 F on Bake function. Crack an egg into a muffin cup. Repeat with the remaining cups. Sprinkle with salt and pepper. Top with cottage cheese. Put the cups in the Air Fryer tray and bake for 8-10 minutes. Remove and sprinkle with paprika to serve.

96. Baja Fish Tacos

Servings: 6 Tacos
Cooking Time: 17 Minutes
Ingredients:
- 1 egg
- 5 ounces (142 g) Mexican beer
- ¾ cup all-purpose flour
- ¾ cup cornstarch
- ¼ teaspoon chili powder
- ½ teaspoon ground cumin
- ½ pound (227 g) cod, cut into large pieces
- 6 corn tortillas
- Cooking spray
- Salsa:
- 1 mango, peeled and diced
- ¼ red bell pepper, diced
- ½ small jalapeño, diced
- ¼ red onion, minced
- Juice of half a lime
- Pinch chopped fresh cilantro
- ¼ teaspoon salt
- ¼ teaspoon ground black pepper

Directions:
1. Spritz the air fryer basket with cooking spray.
2. Whisk the egg with beer in a bowl. Combine the flour, cornstarch, chili powder, and cumin in a separate bowl.
3. Dredge the cod in the egg mixture first, then in the flour mixture to coat well. Shake the excess off.
4. Arrange the cod in the basket and spritz with cooking spray.
5. Put the air fryer basket on the baking pan and slide into Rack Position 2, select Air Fry, set temperature to 380ºF (193ºC) and set time to 17 minutes.
6. Flip the cod halfway through the cooking time.
7. When cooked, the cod should be golden brown and crunchy.
8. Meanwhile, combine the ingredients for the salsa in a small bowl. Stir to mix well.
9. Unfold the tortillas on a clean work surface, then divide the fish on the tortillas and spread the salsa on top. Fold to serve.

97. Egg English Muffin With Bacon

Servings:1

Cooking Time: 10 Minutes

Ingredients:
- 1 egg
- 1 English muffin
- 2 slices of bacon
- Salt and black pepper to taste

Directions:
1. Preheat on Bake function to 395 F. Crack the egg into a ramekin. Place the muffin, egg and bacon in the oven. Cook for 9 minutes. Let cool slightly so you can assemble the sandwich.
2. Cut the muffin in half. Place the egg on one half and season with salt and pepper. Arrange the bacon on top. Top with the other muffin half.

98. Nutmeg Potato Gratin

Servings: 5
Cooking Time: 45 Minutes

Ingredients:
- 5 large potatoes
- ½ cup sour cream
- ½ cup grated cheese
- ½ cup milk
- ½ tsp nutmeg
- Salt and black pepper to taste

Directions:
1. Preheat on Bake function to 375 F, peel and slice the potatoes. In a bowl, combine the sour cream, milk, pepper, salt, and nutmeg. Add in the potato slices and stir to coat them well.
2. Transfer the mixture to an ovenproof casserole. Cook for 15 minutes on Bake function, then sprinkle the cheese on top and cook for 10 minutes. Allow to sit for 10 minutes before serving.

99. Amazing Apple & Brie Sandwich

Servings:1
Cooking Time: 10 Minutes

Ingredients:
- 2 bread slices
- ½ apple, thinly sliced
- 2 tsp butter
- 2 oz brie cheese, thinly sliced

Directions:
1. Spread butter on the outside of the bread slices. Arrange apple slices on the inside of one bread slice. Place brie slices on top of the apple. Top with the other slice of bread. Press Start on the oven and cook for 5 minutes at 350 F on Bake function. Cut diagonally and serve.

100. Creamy Potato Gratin With Nutmeg

Servings:4
Cooking Time: 30 Minutes

Ingredients:
- 1 lb potatoes, peeled and sliced
- ½ cup sour cream
- ½ cup mozzarella cheese, grated
- ½ cup milk
- ½ tsp nutmeg
- Salt and black pepper to taste

Directions:
1. Preheat on Bake function to 390 F. In a bowl, combine sour cream, milk, pepper, salt, and nutmeg. Place the potato slices in the bowl with the milk mixture and stir to coat well.
2. Transfer the mixture to a baking dish and press Start. Cook for 20 minutes, then sprinkle grated cheese on top and cook for 5 more minutes. Serve warm.

101. Fried Eggplant Parmesan With Mozzarella Cheese

Servings:x
Cooking Time:x

Ingredients:
- 1/3 cup (45g) all-purpose flour
- 2 eggs
- 1 (28-ounce/790g) can whole tomatoes
- 2 tablespoons olive oil
- 2 cloves garlic, minced
- 1 medium eggplant (about 1 pound/
- 450g)
- 1 cup (55g) panko breadcrumbs
- 1 cup (60g) finely grated Parmesan cheese
- 1 teaspoon dried oregano
- ½ teaspoon dried oregano
- Pinch red pepper flakes
- 1 cup (115g) shredded mozzarella cheese
- 1 cup (20g) finely grated Parmesan
- 1 teaspoon kosher salt
- ¼ teaspoon freshly ground black pepper
- 1 teaspoon kosher salt
- Cheese

Directions:
1. Slice eggplant crosswise into ½-inch (1cm) slices. Lay slices in single layer on a baking sheet and sprinkle with ½ teaspoon kosher salt. Flip slices and sprinkle with another ½ teaspoon salt. Let rest for 20 minutes while preparing breading.
2. Combine panko, Parmesan, oregano, salt and black pepper in bowl of food processor. Process until finely ground, about 15–20 seconds. Transfer to a shallow dish.
3. Place flour in a second shallow dish. Scramble eggs and 2 tablespoons water in a third shallow dish.
4. Use paper towels or a clean dish towel to dry the eggplant slices, pressing firmly on both sides to remove as much moisture as possible.

5. Working in batches, toss eggplant in flour and shake off any excess. Dip eggplant in egg and allow excess to drain off. Dredge eggplant in panko mixture, ensuring all sides are well crusted. If there are any extra breadcrumbs, reserve them to sprinkle on top of casserole.
6. Place half of eggplant on the air fry rack in a single layer. Reserve remaining eggplant on a dry baking pan.
7. Select AIRFRY/375°F (190°C)/SUPER CONVECTION/20 minutes and press START to preheat oven.
8. Cook in rack position 4 until brown and crispy, about 20 minutes. Repeat with remaining eggplant. 9. While eggplant is cooking, make the sauce.
9. Pour tomatoes and their juices into a large bowl and crush with your hands. Alternatively, blend with an immersion blender or food processor for a smoother sauce.
10. Heat olive oil in a medium saucepan over medium heat. Add minced garlic and cook, stirring constantly, until just golden, about 30 seconds. Add the crushed tomatoes, salt, oregano and red pepper flakes and stir to combine.
11. Simmer sauce for 10 minutes, stirring occasionally. Remove from heat and reserve.

102.Crustless Breakfast Quiche

Servings: 4
Cooking Time: 10 Minutes
Ingredients:
- 6 eggs
- 1 cup cheddar cheese, shredded
- 1/4 cup milk
- 1 shallot, sliced & sautéed
- 3 bacon slices, sautéed & chopped
- 1/8 tsp pepper
- 1/8 tsp kosher salt

Directions:
1. Fit the oven with the rack in position
2. Spray an 8-inch baking dish with cooking spray and set aside.
3. In a bowl, whisk eggs with milk, pepper, and salt.
4. Add cheese, shallot, and bacon and stir well.
5. Pour egg mixture into the prepared baking dish.
6. Set to bake at 375 F for 15 minutes. After 5 minutes place the baking dish in the preheated oven.
7. Serve and enjoy.
- **Nutrition Info:** Calories 301 Fat 22.2 g Carbohydrates 3.7 g Sugar 1.4 g Protein 21.4 g Cholesterol 292 mg

103.Tasty Cheddar Omelet

Servings: 1
Cooking Time: 20 Minutes
Ingredients:
- 2 eggs
- 2 tbsp cheddar cheese, grated
- 1 tsp soy sauce
- ½ onion, sliced
- Salt and black pepper to taste
- 1 tbsp olive oil

Directions:
1. Preheat on Bake function to 350 F. Whisk the eggs with soy sauce, salt, and pepper. Stir in onion. Grease a baking dish with the olive oil and add in the egg mixture. Cook for 10-14 minutes. Top with the grated cheddar cheese and serve.

104.Cheesy Bacon And Egg Wraps

Servings:3
Cooking Time: 10 Minutes
Ingredients:
- 3 corn tortillas
- 3 slices bacon, cut into strips
- 2 scrambled eggs
- 3 tablespoons salsa
- 1 cup grated Pepper Jack cheese
- 3 tablespoons cream cheese, divided
- Cooking spray

Directions:
1. Spritz the air fryer basket with cooking spray.
2. Unfold the tortillas on a clean work surface, divide the bacon and eggs in the middle of the tortillas, then spread with salsa and scatter with cheeses. Fold the tortillas over.
3. Arrange the tortillas in the pan.
4. Put the air fryer basket on the baking pan and slide into Rack Position 2, select Air Fry, set temperature to 390ºF (199ºC) and set time to 10 minutes.
5. Flip the tortillas halfway through the cooking time.
6. When cooking is complete, the cheeses will be melted and the tortillas will be lightly browned.
7. Serve immediately.

105.Delicious French Eggs

Servings: 12
Cooking Time: 10 Minutes
Ingredients:
- 12 eggs
- 1/2 cup heavy cream
- 8 oz parmesan cheese, shredded
- Pepper
- Salt

Directions:
1. Fit the oven with the rack in position

2. Spray 12-cups muffin tin with cooking spray and set aside.
3. Crack each egg into each cup.
4. Divide heavy cream and parmesan cheese evenly into each cup.
5. Season with pepper and salt.
6. Set to bake at 425 F for 15 minutes. After 5 minutes place muffin tin in the preheated oven.
7. Serve and enjoy.
- **Nutrition Info:** Calories 141 Fat 10.3 g Carbohydrates 1.2 g Sugar 0.4 g Protein 11.7 g Cholesterol 184 mg

106.Bourbon Vanilla French Toast

Servings:4
Cooking Time: 6 Minutes
Ingredients:
- 2 large eggs
- 2 tablespoons water
- $^2/_3$ cup whole or 2% milk
- 1 tablespoon butter, melted
- 2 tablespoons bourbon
- 1 teaspoon vanilla extract
- 8 (1-inch-thick) French bread slices
- Cooking spray

Directions:
1. Spray the baking pan with cooking spray.
2. Beat the eggs with the water in a shallow bowl until combined. Add the milk, melted butter, bourbon, and vanilla and stir to mix well.
3. Dredge 4 slices of bread in the batter, turning to coat both sides evenly. Transfer the bread slices to the baking pan.
4. Slide the baking pan into Rack Position 1, select Convection Bake, set temperature to 320ºF (160ºC) and set time to 6 minutes.
5. Flip the slices halfway through the cooking time.
6. When cooking is complete, the bread slices should be nicely browned.
7. Remove from the oven to a plate and serve warm.

107.Paprika Baked Eggs

Servings:6
Cooking Time: 10 Minutes
Ingredients:
- 6 large eggs
- 1 tsp paprika

Directions:
1. Preheat fryer to 300 F. Lay the eggs in the basket and press Start. Cook for 8 minutes on Bake function. Using tongs, dip the eggs in a bowl with icy water. Let sit for 5 minutes before peeling. Slice, sprinkle with paprika, and serve.

108.Fried Cheese Grits

Servings:4
Cooking Time: 11 Minutes
Ingredients:
- $^2/_3$ cup instant grits
- 1 teaspoon salt
- 1 teaspoon freshly ground black pepper
- ¾ cup whole or 2% milk
- 3 ounces (85 g) cream cheese, at room temperature
- 1 large egg, beaten
- 1 tablespoon butter, melted
- 1 cup shredded mild Cheddar cheese
- Cooking spray

Directions:
1. Mix the grits, salt, and black pepper in a large bowl. Add the milk, cream cheese, beaten egg, and melted butter and whisk to combine. Fold in the Cheddar cheese and stir well.
2. Spray the baking pan with cooking spray. Spread the grits mixture into the baking pan.
3. Put the air fryer basket on the baking pan and slide into Rack Position 2, select Air Fry, set temperature to 400ºF (205ºC) and set time to 11 minutes.
4. Stir the mixture halfway through the cooking time.
5. When done, a knife inserted in the center should come out clean.
6. Rest for 5 minutes and serve warm.

109.Easy Cheese Egg Casserole

Servings: 10
Cooking Time: 40 Minutes
Ingredients:
- 12 eggs
- 8 oz cheddar cheese, shredded
- 1/3 cup milk
- 1/4 tsp pepper
- 1 tsp salt

Directions:
1. Fit the oven with the rack in position
2. Spray 9*13-inch casserole dish with cooking spray and set aside.
3. In a bowl, whisk eggs with milk, pepper, and salt.
4. Add shredded cheese and stir well.
5. Pour egg mixture into the prepared casserole dish.
6. Set to bake at 350 F for 45 minutes. After 5 minutes place the casserole dish in the preheated oven.
7. Serve and enjoy.
- **Nutrition Info:** Calories 171 Fat 12.9 g Carbohydrates 1.1 g Sugar 0.9 g Protein 12.6 g Cholesterol 221 mg

110. Breakfast Oatmeal Cake

Servings: 8
Cooking Time: 25 Minutes
Ingredients:
- 2 eggs
- 1 tbsp coconut oil
- 3 tbsp yogurt
- 1/2 tsp baking powder
- 1 tsp cinnamon
- 1 tsp vanilla
- 3 tbsp honey
- 1/2 tsp baking soda
- 1 apple, peel & chopped
- 1 cup oats

Directions:
1. Fit the oven with the rack in position
2. Line baking dish with parchment paper and set aside.
3. Add 3/4 cup oats and remaining ingredients into the blender and blend until smooth.
4. Add remaining oats and stir well.
5. Pour mixture into the prepared baking dish.
6. Set to bake at 350 F for 30 minutes. After 5 minutes place the baking dish in the preheated oven.
7. Slice and serve.
- **Nutrition Info:** Calories 114 Fat 3.6 g Carbohydrates 18.2 g Sugar 10 g Protein 3.2 g Cholesterol 41 mg

111. Peanut Butter And Jelly Banana Boats

Servings: 1
Cooking Time: 15 Minutes
Ingredients:
- 1 banana
- 1/4 cup peanut butter
- 1/4 cup jelly
- 1 tablespoon granola

Directions:
1. Start by preheating toaster oven to 350°F.
2. Slice banana lengthwise and separate slightly.
3. Spread peanut butter and jelly in the gap.
4. Sprinkle granola over the entire banana.
5. Bake for 15 minutes.
- **Nutrition Info:** Calories: 724, Sodium: 327 mg, Dietary Fiber: 9.2 g, Total Fat: 36.6 g, Total Carbs: 102.9 g, Protein: 20.0 g.

112. Cashew Granola With Cranberries

Servings: 6
Cooking Time: 12 Minutes
Ingredients:
- 3 cups old-fashioned rolled oats
- 2 cups raw cashews
- 1 cup unsweetened coconut chips
- ½ cup honey
- ¼ cup vegetable oil
- ⅓ cup packed light brown sugar
- ¼ teaspoon kosher salt
- 1 cup dried cranberries

Directions:
1. In a large bowl, stir together all the ingredients, except for the cranberries. Spread the mixture in the baking pan in an even layer.
2. Slide the baking pan into Rack Position 1, select Convection Bake, set temperature to 325ºF (163ºC) and set time to 12 minutes.
3. After 5 to 6 minutes, remove the pan and stir the granola. Return the pan to the oven and continue cooking.
4. When cooking is complete, remove the pan. Let the granola cool to room temperature. Stir in the cranberries before serving.

113. Basil Dill Egg Muffins

Servings: 6
Cooking Time: 20 Minutes
Ingredients:
- 6 eggs
- 1 tbsp chives, chopped
- 1 tbsp fresh basil, chopped
- 1 tbsp fresh cilantro, chopped
- 1/4 cup mozzarella cheese, grated
- 1 tbsp fresh dill, chopped
- 1 tbsp fresh parsley, chopped
- Pepper
- Salt

Directions:
1. Fit the oven with the rack in position
2. Spray 6-cups muffin tin with cooking spray and set aside.
3. In a bowl, whisk eggs with pepper and salt.
4. Add remaining ingredients and stir well.
5. Pour egg mixture into the prepared muffin tin.
6. Set to bake at 350 F for 25 minutes. After 5 minutes place muffin tin in the preheated oven.
7. Serve and enjoy.
- **Nutrition Info:** Calories 68 Fat 4.6 g Carbohydrates 0.8 g Sugar 0.4 g Protein 6 g Cholesterol 164 mg

114. Nutritious Cinnamon Oat Muffins

Servings: 12
Cooking Time: 30 Minutes
Ingredients:
- 2 cups oat flour
- 1/3 cup coconut oil, melted
- 1/2 cup maple syrup
- 1 cup applesauce
- 1 tsp cinnamon
- 2 tsp baking powder
- 1 tsp vanilla
- 1/4 tsp salt

Directions:

1. Fit the oven with the rack in position
2. Line 12-cups muffin tin with cupcake liners and set aside.
3. In a bowl, add applesauce, cinnamon, vanilla, oil, maple syrup, and salt and stir to combine.
4. Add baking powder and oat flour and stir well.
5. Pour batter into the prepared muffin tin.
6. Set to bake at 350 F for 35 minutes, after 5 minutes, place the muffin tin in the oven.
7. Serve and enjoy.
- **Nutrition Info:** Calories 158 Fat 7.1 g Carbohydrates 22.2 g Sugar 9.9 g Protein 2 g Cholesterol 0 mg

LUNCH RECIPES

115.Air Fryer Marinated Salmon

Servings: 4
Cooking Time: 12 Minutes
Ingredients:
- 4 salmon fillets or 1 1lb fillet cut into 4 pieces
- 1 Tbsp brown sugar
- ½ Tbsp Minced Garlic
- 6 Tbsps Soy Sauce
- ¼ cup Dijon Mustard
- 1 Green onions finely chopped

Directions:
1. Take a bowl and whisk together soy sauce, dijon mustard, brown sugar, and minced garlic. Pour this mixture over salmon fillets, making sure that all the fillets are covered. Refrigerate and marinate for 20-30 minutes.
2. Remove salmon fillets from marinade and place them in greased or lined on the tray in the Instant Pot Duo Crisp Air Fryer basket, close the lid.
3. Select the Air Fry option and Air Fry for around 12 minutes at 400°F.
4. Remove from Instant Pot Duo Crisp Air Fryer and top with chopped green onions.
- **Nutrition Info:** Calories 267, Total Fat 11g, Total Carbs 5g, Protein 37g

116.Barbecue Air Fried Chicken

Servings: 10
Cooking Time: 26 Minutes
Ingredients:
- 1 teaspoon Liquid Smoke
- 2 cloves Fresh Garlic smashed
- 1/2 cup Apple Cider Vinegar
- 3 pounds Chuck Roast well-marbled with intramuscular fat
- 1 Tablespoon Kosher Salt
- 1 Tablespoon Freshly Ground Black Pepper
- 2 teaspoons Garlic Powder
- 1.5 cups Barbecue Sauce
- 1/4 cup Light Brown Sugar + more for sprinkling
- 2 Tablespoons Honey optional and in place of 2 TBL sugar

Directions:
1. Add meat to the Instant Pot Duo Crisp Air Fryer Basket, spreading out the meat.
2. Select the option Air Fry.
3. Close the Air Fryer lid and cook at 300 degrees F for 8 minutes. Pause the Air Fryer and flip meat over after 4 minutes.
4. Remove the lid and baste with more barbecue sauce and sprinkle with a little brown sugar.
5. Again Close the Air Fryer lid and set the temperature at 400°F for 9 minutes. Watch meat though the lid and flip it over after 5 minutes.
- **Nutrition Info:** Calories 360, Total Fat 16g, Total Carbs 27g, Protein 27g

117.Onion Omelet

Servings: 2
Cooking Time: 15 Minutes
Ingredients:
- 4 eggs
- ¼ teaspoon low-sodium soy sauce
- Ground black pepper, as required
- 1 teaspoon butter
- 1 medium yellow onion, sliced
- ¼ cup Cheddar cheese, grated

Directions:
1. In a skillet, melt the butter over medium heat and cook the onion and cook for about 8-10 minutes.
2. Remove from the heat and set aside to cool slightly.
3. Meanwhile, in a bowl, add the eggs, soy sauce and black pepper and beat well.
4. Add the cooked onion and gently, stir to combine.
5. Place the zucchini mixture into a small baking pan.
6. Press "Power Button" of Air Fry Oven and turn the dial to select the "Air Fry" mode.
7. Press the Time button and again turn the dial to set the cooking time to 5 minutes.
8. Now push the Temp button and rotate the dial to set the temperature at 355 degrees F.
9. Press "Start/Pause" button to start.
10. When the unit beeps to show that it is preheated, open the lid.
11. Arrange pan over the "Wire Rack" and insert in the oven.
12. Cut the omelet into 2 portions and serve hot.
- **Nutrition Info:** Calories: 222 Cal Total Fat: 15.4 g Saturated Fat: 6.9 g Cholesterol: 347 mg Sodium: 264 mg Total Carbs: 6.1 g Fiber: 1.2 g Sugar: 3.1 g Protein: 15.3 g

118.Buttermilk Brined Turkey Breast

Servings: 8
Cooking Time: 20 Minutes
Ingredients:
- ¾ cup brine from a can of olives
- 3½ pounds boneless, skinless turkey breast
- 2 fresh thyme sprigs
- 1 fresh rosemary sprig
- ½ cup buttermilk

Directions:
1. Preheat the Air fryer to 350 degree F and grease an Air fryer basket.
2. Mix olive brine and buttermilk in a bowl until well combined.

3. Place the turkey breast, buttermilk mixture and herb sprigs in a resealable plastic bag.
4. Seal the bag and refrigerate for about 12 hours.
5. Remove the turkey breast from bag and arrange the turkey breast into the Air fryer basket.
6. Cook for about 20 minutes, flipping once in between.
7. Dish out the turkey breast onto a cutting board and cut into desired size slices to serve.
- **Nutrition Info:** Calories: 215, Fat: 3.5g, Carbohydrates: 9.4g, Sugar: 7.7g, Protein: 34.4g, Sodium: 2000mg

119. Chicken Wings With Prawn Paste

Servings: 6
Cooking Time: 8 Minutes
Ingredients:
- Corn flour, as required
- 2 pounds mid-joint chicken wings
- 2 tablespoons prawn paste
- 4 tablespoons olive oil
- 1½ teaspoons sugar
- 2 teaspoons sesame oil
- 1 teaspoon Shaoxing wine
- 2 teaspoons fresh ginger juice

Directions:
1. Preheat the Air fryer to 360 degree F and grease an Air fryer basket.
2. Mix all the ingredients in a bowl except wings and corn flour.
3. Rub the chicken wings generously with marinade and refrigerate overnight.
4. Coat the chicken wings evenly with corn flour and keep aside.
5. Set the Air fryer to 390 degree F and arrange the chicken wings in the Air fryer basket.
6. Cook for about 8 minutes and dish out to serve hot.
- **Nutrition Info:** Calories: 416, Fat: 31.5g, Carbohydrates: 11.2g, Sugar: 1.6g, Protein: 24.4g, Sodium: 661mg

120. Easy Turkey Breasts With Basil

Servings: 4
Cooking Time: 10 Minutes
Ingredients:
- 2 tablespoons olive oil
- 2 pounds turkey breasts, bone-in skin-on
- Coarse sea salt and ground black pepper, to taste
- 1 teaspoon fresh basil leaves, chopped
- 2 tablespoons lemon zest, grated

Directions:

1. Rub olive oil on all sides of the turkey breasts; sprinkle with salt, pepper, basil, and lemon zest.
2. Place the turkey breasts skin side up on a parchment-lined cooking basket.
3. Cook in the preheated Air Fryer at 330 degrees F for 30 minutes. Now, turn them over and cook an additional 28 minutes.
4. Serve with lemon wedges, if desired.
- **Nutrition Info:** 416 Calories; 26g Fat; 0g Carbs; 49g Protein; 0g Sugars; 2g Fiber

121. Sweet Potato And Parsnip Spiralized Latkes

Servings: 12
Cooking Time: 20 Minutes
Ingredients:
- 1 medium sweet potato
- 1 large parsnip
- 4 cups water
- 1 egg + 1 egg white
- 2 scallions
- 1/2 teaspoon garlic powder
- 1/2 teaspoon sea salt
- 1/2 teaspoon ground pepper

Directions:
1. Start by spiralizing the sweet potato and parsnip and chopping the scallions, reserving only the green parts.
2. Preheat toaster oven to 425°F.
3. Bring 4 cups of water to a boil. Place all of your noodles in a colander and pour the boiling water over the top, draining well.
4. Let the noodles cool, then grab handfuls and place them in a paper towel; squeeze to remove as much liquid as possible.
5. In a large bowl, beat egg and egg white together. Add noodles, scallions, garlic powder, salt, and pepper, mix well.
6. Prepare a baking sheet; scoop out 1/4 cup of mixture at a time and place on sheet.
7. Slightly press down each scoop with your hands, then bake for 20 minutes, flipping halfway through.
- **Nutrition Info:** Calories: 24, Sodium: 91 mg, Dietary Fiber: 1.0 g, Total Fat: 0.4 g, Total Carbs: 4.3 g, Protein: 0.9 g.

122. Roasted Beet Salad With Oranges & Beet Greens

Servings: 6
Cooking Time: 1-1/2 Hours
Ingredients:
- 6 medium beets with beet greens attached
- 2 large oranges
- 1 small sweet onion, cut into wedges
- 1/3 cup red wine vinegar
- 1/4 cup extra-virgin olive oil
- 2 garlic cloves, minced

- 1/2 teaspoon grated orange peel

Directions:
1. Start by preheating toaster oven to 400°F.
2. Trim leaves from beets and chop, then set aside.
3. Pierce beets with a fork and place in a roasting pan.
4. Roast beets for 1-1/2 hours.
5. Allow beets to cool, peel, then cut into 8 wedges and put into a bowl.
6. Place beet greens in a sauce pan and cover with just enough water to cover. Heat until water boils, then immediately remove from heat.
7. Drain greens and press to remove liquid from greens, then add to beet bowl.
8. Remove peel and pith from orange and segment, adding each segment to the bowl.
9. Add onion to beet mixture. In a separate bowl mix together vinegar, oil, garlic and orange peel.
10. Combine both bowls and toss, sprinkle with salt and pepper.
11. Let stand for an hour before serving.
- **Nutrition Info:** Calories: 214, Sodium: 183 mg, Dietary Fiber: 6.5 g, Total Fat: 8.9 g, Total Carbs: 32.4 g, Protein: 4.7 g.

123.Creamy Green Beans And Tomatoes

Servings: 4
Cooking Time: 20 Minutes
Ingredients:
- 1 pound green beans, trimmed and halved
- ½ pound cherry tomatoes, halved
- 2 tablespoons olive oil
- 1 teaspoon oregano, dried
- 1 teaspoon basil, dried
- Salt and black pepper to the taste
- 1 cup heavy cream
- ½ tablespoon cilantro, chopped

Directions:
1. In your air fryer's pan, combine the green beans with the tomatoes and the other Ingredients:, toss and cook at 360 degrees F for 20 minutes.
2. Divide the mix between plates and serve.
- **Nutrition Info:** Calories 174, fat 5, fiber 7, carbs 11, protein 4

124.Beef Steaks With Beans

Servings: 4
Cooking Time: 10 Minutes
Ingredients:
- 4 beef steaks, trim the fat and cut into strips
- 1 cup green onions, chopped
- 2 cloves garlic, minced
- 1 red bell pepper, seeded and thinly sliced
- 1 can tomatoes, crushed
- 1 can cannellini beans

- 3/4 cup beef broth
- 1/4 teaspoon dried basil
- 1/2 teaspoon cayenne pepper
- 1/2 teaspoon sea salt
- 1/4 teaspoon ground black pepper, or to taste

Directions:
1. Preparing the ingredients. Add the steaks, green onions and garlic to the instant crisp air fryer basket.
2. Air frying. Close air fryer lid. Cook at 390 degrees f for 10 minutes, working in batches.
3. Stir in the remaining ingredients and cook for an additional 5 minutes.
- **Nutrition Info:** Calories 284 Total fat 7.9 g Saturated fat 1.4 g Cholesterol 36 mg Sodium 704 mg Total carbs 46 g Fiber 3.6 g Sugar 5.5 g Protein 17.9 g

125.Pumpkin Pancakes

Servings: 4
Cooking Time: 12 Minutes
Ingredients:
- 1 square puff pastry
- 3 tablespoons pumpkin filling
- 1 small egg, beaten

Directions:
1. Roll out a square of puff pastry and layer it with pumpkin pie filling, leaving about ¼-inch space around the edges.
2. Cut it up into 8 equal sized square pieces and coat the edges with beaten egg.
3. Press "Power Button" of Air Fry Oven and turn the dial to select the "Air Fry" mode.
4. Press the Time button and again turn the dial to set the cooking time to 12 minutes.
5. Now push the Temp button and rotate the dial to set the temperature at 355 degrees F.
6. Press "Start/Pause" button to start.
7. When the unit beeps to show that it is preheated, open the lid.
8. Arrange the squares into a greased "Sheet Pan" and insert in the oven.
9. Serve warm.
- **Nutrition Info:** Calories: 109 Cal Total Fat: 6.7 g Saturated Fat: 1.8 g Cholesterol: 34 mg Sodium: 87 mg Total Carbs: 9.8 g Fiber: 0.5 g Sugar: 2.6 g Protein: 2.4 g

126.Easy Italian Meatballs

Servings: 4
Cooking Time: 13 Minutes
Ingredients:
- 2-lb. lean ground turkey
- ¼ cup onion, minced
- 2 cloves garlic, minced
- 2 tablespoons parsley, chopped
- 2 eggs

- 1½ cup parmesan cheese, grated
- ½ teaspoon red pepper flakes
- ½ teaspoon Italian seasoning Salt and black pepper to taste

Directions:
1. Toss all the meatball Ingredients: in a bowl and mix well.
2. Make small meatballs out this mixture and place them in the air fryer basket.
3. Press "Power Button" of Air Fry Oven and turn the dial to select the "Air Fry" mode.
4. Press the Time button and again turn the dial to set the cooking time to 13 minutes.
5. Now push the Temp button and rotate the dial to set the temperature at 350 degrees F.
6. Once preheated, place the air fryer basket inside and close its lid.
7. Flip the meatballs when cooked halfway through.
8. Serve warm.
- **Nutrition Info:** Calories 472 Total Fat 25.8 g Saturated Fat .4 g Cholesterol 268 mg Sodium 503 mg Total Carbs 1.7 g Fiber 0.3 g Sugar 0.6 g Protein 59.6 g

127.Vegetarian Philly Sandwich

Servings: 2
Cooking Time: 20 Minutes
Ingredients:
- 2 tablespoons olive oil
- 8 ounces sliced portabello mushrooms
- 1 vidalia onion, thinly sliced
- 1 green bell pepper, thinly sliced
- 1 red bell pepper, thinly sliced
- Salt and pepper
- 4 slices 2% provolone cheese
- 4 rolls

Directions:
1. Preheat toaster oven to 475°F.
2. Heat the oil in a medium sauce pan over medium heat.
3. Sauté mushrooms about 5 minutes, then add the onions and peppers and sauté another 10 minutes.
4. Slice rolls lengthwise and divide the vegetables into each roll.
5. Add the cheese and toast until the rolls start to brown and the cheese melts.
- **Nutrition Info:** Calories: 645, Sodium: 916 mg, Dietary Fiber: 7.2 g, Total Fat: 33.3 g, Total Carbs: 61.8 g, Protein: 27.1 g.

128.Air Fried Sausages

Servings: 6
Cooking Time: 13 Minutes
Ingredients:
- 6 sausage
- olive oil spray

Directions:

1. Pour 5 cup of water into Instant Pot Duo Crisp Air Fryer. Place air fryer basket inside the pot, spray inside with nonstick spray and put sausage links inside.
2. Close the Air Fryer lid and steam for about 5 minutes.
3. Remove the lid once done. Spray links with olive oil and close air crisp lid.
4. Set to air crisp at 400°F for 8 min flipping halfway through so both sides get browned.
- **Nutrition Info:** Calories 267, Total Fat 23g, Total Carbs 2g, Protein 13g

129.Chicken Potato Bake

Servings: 4
Cooking Time: 25 Minutes
Ingredients:
- 4 potatoes, diced
- 1 tablespoon garlic, minced
- 1.5 tablespoons olive oil
- 1/8 teaspoon salt
- 1/8 teaspoon pepper
- 1.5 lbs. boneless skinless chicken
- 3/4 cup mozzarella cheese, shredded
- parsley chopped

Directions:
1. Toss chicken and potatoes with all the spices and oil in a baking pan.
2. Drizzle the cheese on top of the chicken and potato.
3. Press "Power Button" of Air Fry Oven and turn the dial to select the "Bake" mode.
4. Press the Time button and again turn the dial to set the cooking time to 25 minutes.
5. Now push the Temp button and rotate the dial to set the temperature at 375 degrees F.
6. Once preheated, place the baking pan inside and close its lid.
7. Serve warm.
- **Nutrition Info:** Calories 695 Total Fat 17.5 g Saturated Fat 4.8 g Cholesterol 283 mg Sodium 355 mg Total Carbs 26.4 g Fiber 1.8 g Sugar 0.8 g Protein 117.4 g

130.Seven-layer Tostadas

Servings: 6
Cooking Time: 5 Minutes
Ingredients:
- 1 (16-ounce) can refried pinto beans
- 1-1/2 cups guacamole
- 1 cup light sour cream
- 1/2 teaspoon taco seasoning
- 1 cup shredded Mexican cheese blend
- 1 cup chopped tomatoes
- 1/2 cup thinly sliced green onions
- 1/2 cup sliced black olives
- 6-8 whole wheat flour tortillas small enough to fit in your oven
- Olive oil

Directions:

1. Start by placing baking sheet into toaster oven while preheating it to 450°F. Remove pan and drizzle with olive oil.
2. Place tortillas on pan and cook in oven until they are crisp, turn at least once, this should take about 5 minutes or less.
3. In a medium bowl, mash refried beans to break apart any chunks, then microwave for 2 1/2 minutes.
4. Stir taco seasoning into the sour cream. Chop vegetables and halve olives.
5. Top tortillas with ingredients in this order: refried beans, guacamole, sour cream, shredded cheese, tomatoes, onions, and olives.
- **Nutrition Info:** Calories: 657, Sodium: 581 mg, Dietary Fiber: 16.8 g, Total Fat: 31.7 g, Total Carbs: 71.3 g, Protein: 28.9 g.

131.Pork Stew

Servings: 4
Cooking Time: 12 Minutes
Ingredients:

- 2 lb. pork stew meat; cubed
- 1 eggplant; cubed
- ½ cup beef stock
- 2 zucchinis; cubed
- ½ tsp. smoked paprika
- Salt and black pepper to taste.
- A handful cilantro; chopped.

Directions:

1. In a pan that fits your air fryer, mix all the ingredients, toss, introduce in your air fryer and cook at 370°F for 30 minutes
2. Divide into bowls and serve right away.
- **Nutrition Info:** Calories: 245; Fat: 12g; Fiber: 2g; Carbs: 5g; Protein: 14g

132.Chili Chicken Sliders

Servings: 4
Cooking Time: 10 Minutes
Ingredients:

- 1/3 teaspoon paprika
- 1/3 cup scallions, peeled and chopped
- 3 cloves garlic, peeled and minced
- 1 teaspoon ground black pepper, or to taste
- 1/2 teaspoon fresh basil, minced
- 1 ½ cups chicken,minced
- 1 ½ tablespoons coconut aminos
- 1/2 teaspoon grated fresh ginger
- 1/2 tablespoon chili sauce
- 1 teaspoon salt

Directions:

1. Thoroughly combine all ingredients in a mixing dish. Then, form into 4 patties.
2. Cook in the preheated Air Fryer for 18 minutes at 355 degrees F.
3. Garnish with toppings of choice.

- **Nutrition Info:** 366 Calories; 6g Fat; 4g Carbs; 66g Protein; 3g Sugars; 9g Fiber

133.Maple Chicken Thighs

Servings: 4
Cooking Time: 30 Minutes
Ingredients:

- 4 large chicken thighs, bone-in
- 2 tablespoons French mustard
- 2 tablespoons Dijon mustard
- 1 clove minced garlic
- 1/2 teaspoon dried marjoram
- 2 tablespoons maple syrup

Directions:

1. Mix chicken with everything in a bowl and coat it well.
2. Place the chicken along with its marinade in the baking pan.
3. Press "Power Button" of Air Fry Oven and turn the dial to select the "Bake" mode.
4. Press the Time button and again turn the dial to set the cooking time to 30 minutes.
5. Now push the Temp button and rotate the dial to set the temperature at 370 degrees F.
6. Once preheated, place the baking pan inside and close its lid.
7. Serve warm.
- **Nutrition Info:** Calories 301 Total Fat 15.8 g Saturated Fat 2.7 g Cholesterol 75 mg Sodium 189 mg Total Carbs 31.7 g Fiber 0.3 g Sugar 0.1 g Protein 28.2 g

134.Chicken & Rice Casserole

Servings: 6
Cooking Time: 40 Minutes
Ingredients:

- 2 lbs. bone-in chicken thighs
- Salt and black pepper
- 1 teaspoon olive oil
- 5 cloves garlic, chopped
- 2 large onions, chopped
- 2 large red bell peppers, chopped
- 1 tablespoon sweet Hungarian paprika
- 1 teaspoon hot Hungarian paprika
- 2 tablespoons tomato paste
- 2 cups chicken broth
- 3 cups brown rice, thawed
- 2 tablespoons parsley, chopped
- 6 tablespoons sour cream

Directions:

1. Mix broth, tomato paste, and all the spices in a bowl.
2. Add chicken and mix well to coat.
3. Spread the rice in a casserole dish and add chicken along with its marinade.
4. Top the casserole with the rest of the Ingredients:.
5. Press "Power Button" of Air Fry Oven and turn the dial to select the "Bake" mode.

6. Press the Time button and again turn the dial to set the cooking time to 40 minutes.
7. Now push the Temp button and rotate the dial to set the temperature at 350 degrees F.
8. Once preheated, place the baking pan inside and close its lid.
9. Serve warm.
- **Nutrition Info:** Calories 440 Total Fat 7.9 g Saturated Fat 1.8 g Cholesterol 5 mg Sodium 581 mg Total Carbs 21.8 g Sugar 7.1 g Fiber 2.6 g Protein 37.2 g

135.Coriander Artichokes(3)

Servings: 4
Cooking Time: 12 Minutes
Ingredients:
- 12 oz. artichoke hearts
- 1 tbsp. lemon juice
- 1 tsp. coriander, ground
- ½ tsp. cumin seeds
- ½ tsp. olive oil
- Salt and black pepper to taste.

Directions:
1. In a pan that fits your air fryer, mix all the ingredients, toss, introduce the pan in the fryer and cook at 370°F for 15 minutes
2. Divide the mix between plates and serve as a side dish.
- **Nutrition Info:** Calories: 200; Fat: 7g; Fiber: 2g; Carbs: 5g; Protein: 8g

136.Turkey And Mushroom Stew

Servings: 4
Cooking Time: 12 Minutes
Ingredients:
- ½ lb. brown mushrooms; sliced
- 1 turkey breast, skinless, boneless; cubed and browned
- ¼ cup tomato sauce
- 1 tbsp. parsley; chopped.
- Salt and black pepper to taste.

Directions:
1. In a pan that fits your air fryer, mix the turkey with the mushrooms, salt, pepper and tomato sauce, toss, introduce in the fryer and cook at 350°F for 25 minutes
2. Divide into bowls and serve for lunch with parsley sprinkled on top.
- **Nutrition Info:** Calories: 220; Fat: 12g; Fiber: 2g; Carbs: 5g; Protein: 12g

137.Juicy Turkey Burgers

Servings: 8
Cooking Time: 25 Minutes
Ingredients:
- 1 lb ground turkey 85% lean / 15% fat
- ¼ cup unsweetened apple sauce
- ½ onion grated
- 1 Tbsp ranch seasoning
- 2 tsp Worcestershire Sauce
- 1 tsp minced garlic
- ¼ cup plain breadcrumbs
- Salt and pepper to taste

Directions:
1. Combine the onion, ground turkey, unsweetened apple sauce, minced garlic, breadcrumbs, ranch seasoning, Worchestire sauce, and salt and pepper. Mix them with your hands until well combined. Form 4 equally sized hamburger patties with them.
2. Place these burgers in the refrigerator for about 30 minutes to have them firm up a bit.
3. While preparing for cooking, select the Air Fry option. Set the temperature of 360°F and the cook time as required. Press start to begin preheating.
4. Once the preheating temperature is reached, place the burgers on the tray in the Air fryer basket, making sure they don't overlap or touch. Cook on for 15 minutes
5. flipping halfway through.
- **Nutrition Info:** Calories 183, Total Fat 3g, Total Carbs 11g, Protein 28g

138.Rosemary Lemon Chicken

Servings: 8
Cooking Time: 45 Minutes
Ingredients:
- 4-lb. chicken, cut into pieces
- Salt and black pepper, to taste
- Flour for dredging 3 tablespoons olive oil
- 1 large onion, sliced
- Peel of ½ lemon
- 2 large garlic cloves, minced
- 1 1/2 teaspoons rosemary leaves
- 1 tablespoon honey
- 1/4 cup lemon juice
- 1 cup chicken broth

Directions:
1. Dredges the chicken through the flour then place in the baking pan.
2. Whisk broth with the rest of the Ingredients: in a bowl.
3. Pour this mixture over the dredged chicken in the pan.
4. Press "Power Button" of Air Fry Oven and turn the dial to select the "Bake" mode.
5. Press the Time button and again turn the dial to set the cooking time to 45 minutes.
6. Now push the Temp button and rotate the dial to set the temperature at 400 degrees F.
7. Once preheated, place the baking pan inside and close its lid.
8. Baste the chicken with its sauce every 15 minutes.
9. Serve warm.
- **Nutrition Info:** Calories 405 Total Fat 22.7 g Saturated Fat 6.1 g Cholesterol 4 mg

Sodium 227 mg Total Carbs 26.1 g Fiber 1.4 g Sugar 0.9 g Protein 45.2 g

139.Turkey-stuffed Peppers

Servings: 6
Cooking Time: 35 Minutes
Ingredients:

- 1 pound lean ground turkey
- 1 tablespoon olive oil
- 2 cloves garlic, minced
- 1/3 onion, minced
- 1 tablespoon cilantro (optional)
- 1 teaspoon garlic powder
- 1 teaspoon cumin powder
- 1/2 teaspoon salt
- Pepper to taste
- 3 large red bell peppers
- 1 cup chicken broth
- 1/4 cup tomato sauce
- 1-1/2 cups cooked brown rice
- 1/4 cup shredded cheddar
- 6 green onions

Directions:

1. Start by preheating toaster oven to 400°F.
2. Heat a skillet on medium heat.
3. Add olive oil to the skillet, then mix in onion and garlic.
4. Sauté for about 5 minutes, or until the onion starts to look opaque.
5. Add the turkey to the skillet and season with cumin, garlic powder, salt, and pepper.
6. Brown the meat until thoroughly cooked, then mix in chicken broth and tomato sauce.
7. Reduce heat and simmer for about 5 minutes, stirring occasionally.
8. Add the brown rice and continue stirring until it is evenly spread through the mix.
9. Cut the bell peppers lengthwise down the middle and remove all of the seeds.
10. Grease a pan or line it with parchment paper and lay all peppers in the pan with the outside facing down.
11. Spoon the meat mixture evenly into each pepper and use the back of the spoon to level.
12. Bake for 30 minutes.
13. Remove pan from oven and sprinkle cheddar over each pepper, then put it back in for another 3 minutes, or until the cheese is melted.
14. While the cheese melts, dice the green onions. Remove pan from oven and sprinkle onions over each pepper and serve.
- **Nutrition Info:** Calories: 394, Sodium: 493 mg, Dietary Fiber: 4.1 g, Total Fat: 12.9 g, Total Carbs: 44.4 g, Protein: 27.7 g.

140.Green Bean Casserole(2)

Servings: 4

Cooking Time: 12 Minutes
Ingredients:

- 1 lb. fresh green beans, edges trimmed
- ½ oz. pork rinds, finely ground
- 1 oz. full-fat cream cheese
- ½ cup heavy whipping cream.
- ¼ cup diced yellow onion
- ½ cup chopped white mushrooms
- ½ cup chicken broth
- 4 tbsp. unsalted butter.
- ¼ tsp. xanthan gum

Directions:

1. In a medium skillet over medium heat, melt the butter. Sauté the onion and mushrooms until they become soft and fragrant, about 3–5 minutes.
2. Add the heavy whipping cream, cream cheese and broth to the pan. Whisk until smooth. Bring to a boil and then reduce to a simmer. Sprinkle the xanthan gum into the pan and remove from heat
3. Chop the green beans into 2-inch pieces and place into a 4-cup round baking dish. Pour the sauce mixture over them and stir until coated. Top the dish with ground pork rinds. Place into the air fryer basket
4. Adjust the temperature to 320 Degrees F and set the timer for 15 minutes. Top will be golden and green beans fork tender when fully cooked. Serve warm.
- **Nutrition Info:** Calories: 267; Protein: 6g; Fiber: 2g; Fat: 24g; Carbs: 7g

141.Turkey Meatloaf

Servings: 4
Cooking Time: 20 Minutes
Ingredients:

- 1 pound ground turkey
- 1 cup kale leaves, trimmed and finely chopped
- 1 cup onion, chopped
- ½ cup fresh breadcrumbs
- 1 cup Monterey Jack cheese, grated
- 2 garlic cloves, minced
- ¼ cup salsa verde
- 1 teaspoon red chili powder
- ½ teaspoon ground cumin
- ½ teaspoon dried oregano, crushed
- Salt and ground black pepper, as required

Directions:

1. Preheat the Air fryer to 400 degree F and grease an Air fryer basket.
2. Mix all the ingredients in a bowl and divide the turkey mixture into 4 equal-sized portions.
3. Shape each into a mini loaf and arrange the loaves into the Air fryer basket.
4. Cook for about 20 minutes and dish out to serve warm.

- **Nutrition Info:** Calories: 435, Fat: 23.1g, Carbohydrates: 18.1g, Sugar: 3.6g, Protein: 42.2g, Sodium: 641mg

142.Okra And Green Beans Stew

Servings: 4
Cooking Time: 12 Minutes
Ingredients:
- 1 lb. green beans; halved
- 4 garlic cloves; minced
- 1 cup okra
- 3 tbsp. tomato sauce
- 1 tbsp. thyme; chopped.
- Salt and black pepper to taste.

Directions:
1. In a pan that fits your air fryer, mix all the ingredients, toss, introduce the pan in the air fryer and cook at 370°F for 15 minutes
2. Divide the stew into bowls and serve.
- **Nutrition Info:** Calories: 183; Fat: 5g; Fiber: 2g; Carbs: 4g; Protein: 8g

143.Kale And Pine Nuts

Servings: 4
Cooking Time: 12 Minutes
Ingredients:
- 10 cups kale; torn
- 1/3 cup pine nuts
- 2 tbsp. lemon zest; grated
- 1 tbsp. lemon juice
- 2 tbsp. olive oil
- Salt and black pepper to taste.

Directions:
1. In a pan that fits the air fryer, combine all the ingredients, toss, introduce the pan in the machine and cook at 380°F for 15 minutes
2. Divide between plates and serve as a side dish.
- **Nutrition Info:** Calories: 121; Fat: 9g; Fiber: 2g; Carbs: 4g; Protein: 5g

144.Simple Turkey Breast

Servings: 10
Cooking Time: 40 Minutes
Ingredients:
- 1: 8-poundsbone-in turkey breast
- Salt and black pepper, as required
- 2 tablespoons olive oil

Directions:
1. Preheat the Air fryer to 360 degree F and grease an Air fryer basket.
2. Season the turkey breast with salt and black pepper and drizzle with oil.
3. Arrange the turkey breast into the Air Fryer basket, skin side down and cook for about 20 minutes.
4. Flip the side and cook for another 20 minutes.

5. Dish out in a platter and cut into desired size slices to serve.
- **Nutrition Info:** Calories: 719, Fat: 35.9g, Carbohydrates: 0g, Sugar: 0g, Protein: 97.2g, Sodium: 386mg

145.Coriander Potatoes

Servings: 4
Cooking Time: 25 Minutes
Ingredients:
- 1 pound gold potatoes, peeled and cut into wedges
- Salt and black pepper to the taste
- 1 tablespoon tomato sauce
- 2 tablespoons coriander, chopped
- ½ teaspoon garlic powder
- 1 teaspoon chili powder
- 1 tablespoon olive oil

Directions:
1. In a bowl, combine the potatoes with the tomato sauce and the other Ingredients:, toss, and transfer to the air fryer's basket.
2. Cook at 370 degrees F for 25 minutes, divide between plates and serve as a side dish.
- **Nutrition Info:** Calories 210, fat 5, fiber 7, carbs 12, protein 5

146.Roasted Mini Peppers

Servings: 6
Cooking Time: 15 Minutes
Ingredients:
- 1 bag mini bell peppers
- Cooking spray
- Salt and pepper to taste

Directions:
1. Start by preheating toaster oven to 400°F.
2. Wash and dry the peppers, then place flat on a baking sheet.
3. Spray peppers with cooking spray and sprinkle with salt and pepper.
4. Roast for 15 minutes.
- **Nutrition Info:** Calories: 19, Sodium: 2 mg, Dietary Fiber: 1.3 g, Total Fat: 0.3 g, Total Carbs: 3.6 g, Protein: 0.6 g.

147.Okra Casserole

Servings: 4
Cooking Time: 12 Minutes
Ingredients:
- 2 red bell peppers; cubed
- 2 tomatoes; chopped.
- 3 garlic cloves; minced
- 3 cups okra
- ½ cup cheddar; shredded
- ¼ cup tomato puree
- 1 tbsp. cilantro; chopped.
- 1 tsp. olive oil
- 2 tsp. coriander, ground

- Salt and black pepper to taste.

Directions:

1. Grease a heat proof dish that fits your air fryer with the oil, add all the ingredients except the cilantro and the cheese and toss them really gently
2. Sprinkle the cheese and the cilantro on top, introduce the dish in the fryer and cook at 390°F for 20 minutes.
3. Divide between plates and serve for lunch.
- **Nutrition Info:** Calories: 221; Fat: 7g; Fiber: 2g; Carbs: 4g; Protein: 9g

148. Tomato Frittata

Servings: 2
Cooking Time: 30 Minutes
Ingredients:

- 4 eggs
- ¼ cup onion, chopped
- ½ cup tomatoes, chopped
- ½ cup milk
- 1 cup Gouda cheese, shredded
- Salt, as required

Directions:

1. In a small baking pan, add all the ingredients and mix well.
2. Press "Power Button" of Air Fry Oven and turn the dial to select the "Air Fry" mode.
3. Press the Time button and again turn the dial to set the cooking time to 30 minutes.
4. Now push the Temp button and rotate the dial to set the temperature at 340 degrees F.
5. Press "Start/Pause" button to start.
6. When the unit beeps to show that it is preheated, open the lid.
7. Arrange the baking pan over the "Wire Rack" and insert in the oven.
8. Cut into 2 wedges and serve.
- **Nutrition Info:** Calories: 247 Cal Total Fat: 16.1 g Saturated Fat: 7.5 g Cholesterol: 332 mg Sodium: 417 mg Total Carbs: 7.30 g Fiber: 0.9 g Sugar: 5.2 g Protein: 18.6 g

149. Butter Fish With Sake And Miso

Servings: 4
Cooking Time: 11 Minutes
Ingredients:

- 4 (7-ounce) pieces of butter fish
- 1/3 cup sake
- 1/3 cup mirin
- 2/3 cup sugar
- 1 cup white miso

Directions:

1. Start by combining sake, mirin, and sugar in a sauce pan and bring to a boil.
2. Allow to boil for 5 minutes, then reduce heat and simmer for another 10 minutes.
3. Remove from heat completely and mix in miso.

4. Marinate the fish in the mixture for as long as possible, up to 3 days if possible.
5. Preheat toaster oven to 450°F and bake fish for 8 minutes.
6. Switch your setting to Broil and broil another 2-3 minutes, until the sauce is caramelized.
- **Nutrition Info:** Calories: 529, Sodium: 2892 mg, Dietary Fiber: 3.7 g, Total Fat: 5.8 g, Total Carbs: 61.9 g, Protein: 53.4 g.

150. Fried Paprika Tofu

Servings:
Cooking Time: 12 Minutes
Ingredients:

- 1 block extra firm tofu; pressed to remove excess water and cut into cubes
- 1/4 cup cornstarch
- 1 tablespoon smoked paprika
- salt and pepper to taste

Directions:

1. Line the Air Fryer basket with aluminum foil and brush with oil. Preheat the Air Fryer to 370 - degrees Fahrenheit.
2. Mix all ingredients in a bowl. Toss to combine. Place in the Air Fryer basket and cook for 12 minutes.

151. Roasted Grape And Goat Cheese Crostinis

Servings: 10
Cooking Time: 5 Minutes
Ingredients:

- 1 pound seedless red grapes
- 1 teaspoon chopped rosemary
- 4 tablespoons olive oil
- 1 rustic French baguette
- 1 cup sliced shallots
- 2 tablespoons unsalted butter
- 8 ounces goat cheese
- 1 tablespoon honey

Directions:

1. Start by preheating toaster oven to 400°F.
2. Toss grapes, rosemary, and 1 tablespoon of olive oil in a large bowl.
3. Transfer to a roasting pan and roast for 20 minutes.
4. Remove the pan from the oven and set aside to cool.
5. Slice the baguette into 1/2-inch-thick pieces.
6. Brush each slice with olive oil and place on baking sheet.
7. Bake for 8 minutes, then remove from oven and set aside.
8. In a medium skillet add butter and one tablespoon of olive oil.
9. Add shallots and sauté for about 10 minutes.

10. Mix goat cheese and honey in a medium bowl, then add contents of shallot pan and mix thoroughly.
11. Spread shallot mixture onto baguette, top with grapes, and serve.
- **Nutrition Info:** Calories: 238, Sodium: 139 mg, Dietary Fiber: 0.6 g, Total Fat: 16.3 g, Total Carbs: 16.4 g, Protein: 8.4 g.

152. Chicken Breast With Rosemary

Servings: 4
Cooking Time: 60 Minutes
Ingredients:
- 4 bone-in chicken breast halves
- 3 tablespoons softened butter
- 1/2 teaspoon salt
- 1/4 teaspoon pepper
- 1 tablespoon rosemary
- 1 tablespoon extra-virgin olive oil

Directions:
1. Start by preheating toaster oven to 400°F.
2. Mix butter, salt, pepper, and rosemary in a bowl.
3. Coat chicken with the butter mixture and place in a shallow pan.
4. Drizzle oil over chicken and roast for 25 minutes.
5. Flip chicken and roast for another 20 minutes.
6. Flip chicken one more time and roast for a final 15 minutes.
- **Nutrition Info:** Calories: 392, Sodium: 551 mg, Dietary Fiber: 0 g, Total Fat: 18.4 g, Total Carbs: 0.6 g, Protein: 55.4 g.

153. Herb-roasted Chicken Tenders

Servings: 2
Cooking Time: 10 Minutes
Ingredients:
- 7 ounces chicken tenders
- 1 tablespoon olive oil
- 1/2 teaspoon Herbes de Provence
- 2 tablespoons Dijon mustard
- 1 tablespoon honey
- Salt and pepper

Directions:
1. Start by preheating toaster oven to 450°F.
2. Brush bottom of pan with 1/2 tablespoon olive oil.
3. Season the chicken with herbs, salt, and pepper.
4. Place the chicken in a single flat layer in the pan and drizzle the remaining olive oil over it.
5. Bake for about 10 minutes.
6. While the chicken is baking, mix together the mustard and honey for a tasty condiment.

- **Nutrition Info:** Calories: 297, Sodium: 268 mg, Dietary Fiber: 0.8 g, Total Fat: 15.5 g, Total Carbs: 9.6 g, Protein: 29.8 g.

154. Deviled Chicken

Servings: 8
Cooking Time: 40 Minutes
Ingredients:
- 2 tablespoons butter
- 2 cloves garlic, chopped
- 1 cup Dijon mustard
- 1/2 teaspoon cayenne pepper
- 1 1/2 cups panko breadcrumbs
- 3/4 cup Parmesan, freshly grated
- 1/4 cup chives, chopped
- 2 teaspoons paprika
- 8 small bone-in chicken thighs, skin removed

Directions:
1. Toss the chicken thighs with crumbs, cheese, chives, butter, and spices in a bowl and mix well to coat.
2. Transfer the chicken along with its spice mix to a baking pan.
3. Press "Power Button" of Air Fry Oven and turn the dial to select the "Air Fry" mode.
4. Press the Time button and again turn the dial to set the cooking time to 40 minutes.
5. Now push the Temp button and rotate the dial to set the temperature at 350 degrees F.
6. Once preheated, place the baking pan inside and close its lid.
7. Serve warm.
- **Nutrition Info:** Calories 380 Total Fat 20 g Saturated Fat 5 g Cholesterol 151 mg Sodium 686 mg Total Carbs 33 g Fiber 1 g Sugar 1.2 g Protein 21 g

155. Easy Prosciutto Grilled Cheese

Servings: 1
Cooking Time: 5 Minutes
Ingredients:
- 2 slices muenster cheese
- 2 slices white bread
- Four thinly-shaved pieces of prosciutto
- 1 tablespoon sweet and spicy pickles

Directions:
1. Set toaster oven to the Toast setting.
2. Place one slice of cheese on each piece of bread.
3. Put prosciutto on one slice and pickles on the other.
4. Transfer to a baking sheet and toast for 4 minutes or until the cheese is melted.
5. Combine the sides, cut, and serve.
- **Nutrition Info:** Calories: 460, Sodium: 2180 mg, Dietary Fiber: 0 g, Total Fat: 25.2 g, Total Carbs: 11.9 g, Protein: 44.2 g.

156.Skinny Black Bean Flautas

Servings: 10
Cooking Time: 25 Minutes
Ingredients:
- 2 (15-ounce) cans black beans
- 1 cup shredded cheddar
- 1 (4-ounce) can diced green chilies
- 2 teaspoons taco seasoning
- 10 (8-inch) whole wheat flour tortillas
- Olive oil

Directions:
1. Start by preheating toaster oven to 350°F.
2. Drain black beans and mash in a medium bowl with a fork.
3. Mix in cheese, chilies, and taco seasoning until all ingredients are thoroughly combined.
4. Evenly spread the mixture over each tortilla and wrap tightly.
5. Brush each side lightly with olive oil and place on a baking sheet.
6. Bake for 12 minutes, turn, and bake for another 13 minutes.
- **Nutrition Info:** Calories: 367, Sodium: 136 mg, Dietary Fiber: 14.4 g, Total Fat: 2.8 g, Total Carbs: 64.8 g, Protein: 22.6 g.

157.Lime And Mustard Marinated Chicken

Servings: 4
Cooking Time: 10 Minutes
Ingredients:
- 1/2 teaspoon stone-ground mustard
- 1/2 teaspoon minced fresh oregano
- 1/3 cup freshly squeezed lime juice
- 2 small-sized chicken breasts, skin-on
- 1 teaspoon kosher salt
- 1teaspoon freshly cracked mixed peppercorns

Directions:
1. Preheat your Air Fryer to 345 degrees F.
2. Toss all of the above ingredients in a medium-sized mixing dish; allow it to marinate overnight.
3. Cook in the preheated Air Fryer for 26 minutes.
- **Nutrition Info:** 255 Calories; 15g Fat; 7g Carbs; 33g Protein; 8g Sugars; 3g Fiber

158.Glazed Lamb Chops

Servings: 4
Cooking Time: 15 Minutes
Ingredients:
- 1 tablespoon Dijon mustard
- ½ tablespoon fresh lime juice
- 1 teaspoon honey
- ½ teaspoon olive oil
- Salt and ground black pepper, as required
- 4 (4-ounce) lamb loin chops

Directions:

1. In a black pepper large bowl, mix together the mustard, lemon juice, oil, honey, salt, and black pepper.
2. Add the chops and coat with the mixture generously.
3. Place the chops onto the greased "Sheet Pan".
4. Press "Power Button" of Ninja Foodi Digital Air Fry Oven and turn the dial to select the "Air Bake" mode.
5. Press the Time button and again turn the dial to set the cooking time to 15 minutes.
6. Now push the Temp button and rotate the dial to set the temperature at 390 degrees F.
7. Press "Start/Pause" button to start.
8. When the unit beeps to show that it is preheated, open the lid.
9. Insert the "Sheet Pan" in oven.
10. Flip the chops once halfway through.
11. Serve hot.
- **Nutrition Info:** Calories: 224 kcal Total Fat: 9.1 g Saturated Fat: 3.1 g Cholesterol: 102 mg Sodium: 169 mg Total Carbs: 1.7 g Fiber: 0.1 g Sugar: 1.5 g Protein: 32 g

159.Beer Coated Duck Breast

Servings: 2
Cooking Time: 20 Minutes
Ingredients:
- 1 tablespoon fresh thyme, chopped
- 1 cup beer
- 1: 10½-ouncesduck breast
- 6 cherry tomatoes
- 1 tablespoon olive oil
- 1 teaspoon mustard
- Salt and ground black pepper, as required
- 1 tablespoon balsamic vinegar

Directions:
1. Preheat the Air fryer to 390 degree F and grease an Air fryer basket.
2. Mix the olive oil, mustard, thyme, beer, salt, and black pepper in a bowl.
3. Coat the duck breasts generously with marinade and refrigerate, covered for about 4 hours.
4. Cover the duck breasts and arrange into the Air fryer basket.
5. Cook for about 15 minutes and remove the foil from breast.
6. Set the Air fryer to 355 degree F and place the duck breast and tomatoes into the Air Fryer basket.
7. Cook for about 5 minutes and dish out the duck breasts and cherry tomatoes.
8. Drizzle with vinegar and serve immediately.
- **Nutrition Info:** Calories: 332, Fat: 13.7g, Carbohydrates: 9.2g, Sugar: 2.5g, Protein: 34.6g, Sodium: 88mg

160. Duck Breast With Figs

Servings: 2
Cooking Time: 45 Minutes
Ingredients:
- 1 pound boneless duck breast
- 6 fresh figs, halved
- 1 tablespoon fresh thyme, chopped
- 2 cups fresh pomegranate juice
- 2 tablespoons lemon juice
- 3 tablespoons brown sugar
- 1 teaspoon olive oil
- Salt and black pepper, as required

Directions:
1. Preheat the Air fryer to 400 degree F and grease an Air fryer basket.
2. Put the pomegranate juice, lemon juice, and brown sugar in a medium saucepan over medium heat.
3. Bring to a boil and simmer on low heat for about 25 minutes.
4. Season the duck breasts generously with salt and black pepper.
5. Arrange the duck breasts into the Air fryer basket, skin side up and cook for about 14 minutes, flipping once in between.
6. Dish out the duck breasts onto a cutting board for about 10 minutes.
7. Meanwhile, put the figs, olive oil, salt, and black pepper in a bowl until well mixed.
8. Set the Air fryer to 400 degree F and arrange the figs into the Air fryer basket.
9. Cook for about 5 more minutes and dish out in a platter.
10. Put the duck breast with the roasted figs and drizzle with warm pomegranate juice mixture.
11. Garnish with fresh thyme and serve warm.
- **Nutrition Info:** Calories: 699, Fat: 12.1g, Carbohydrates: 90g, Sugar: 74g, Protein: 519g, Sodium: 110mg

161. Nutmeg Chicken Thighs

Servings: 4
Cooking Time: 10 Minutes
Ingredients:
- 2 lb. chicken thighs
- 2 tbsp. olive oil
- ½ tsp. nutmeg, ground
- A pinch of salt and black pepper

Directions:
1. Season the chicken thighs with salt and pepper and rub with the rest of the ingredients
2. Put the chicken thighs in air fryer's basket, cook at 360°F for 15 minutes on each side, divide between plates and serve.
- **Nutrition Info:** Calories: 271; Fat: 12g; Fiber: 4g; Carbs: 6g; Protein: 13g

162. Sweet Potato Chips

Servings: 2
Cooking Time: 40 Minutes
Ingredients:
- 2 sweet potatoes
- Salt and pepper to taste
- Olive oil
- Cinnamon

Directions:
1. Start by preheating toaster oven to 400°F.
2. Cut off each end of potato and discard.
3. Cut potatoes into 1/2-inch slices.
4. Brush a pan with olive oil and lay potato slices flat on the pan.
5. Bake for 20 minutes, then flip and bake for another 20.
- **Nutrition Info:** Calories: 139, Sodium: 29 mg, Dietary Fiber: 8.2 g, Total Fat: 0.5 g, Total Carbs: 34.1 g, Protein: 1.9 g.

163. Roasted Stuffed Peppers

Servings: 4
Cooking Time: 20 Minutes
Ingredients:
- 4 ounces shredded cheddar cheese
- ½ tsp. Pepper
- ½ tsp. Salt
- 1 tsp. Worcestershire sauce
- ½ c. Tomato sauce
- 8 ounces lean ground beef
- 1 tsp. Olive oil
- 1 minced garlic clove
- ½ chopped onion
- 2 green peppers

Directions:
1. Preparing the ingredients. Ensure your instant crisp air fryer is preheated to 390 degrees. Spray with olive oil.
2. Cut stems off bell peppers and remove seeds. Cook in boiling salted water for 3 minutes.
3. Sauté garlic and onion together in a skillet until golden in color.
4. Take skillet off the heat. Mix pepper, salt, Worcestershire sauce, ¼ cup of tomato sauce, half of cheese and beef together.
5. Divide meat mixture into pepper halves. Top filled peppers with remaining cheese and tomato sauce.
6. Place filled peppers in the instant crisp air fryer.
7. Air frying. Close air fryer lid. Set temperature to 390°f, and set time to 20 minutes, bake 15-20 minutes.
- **Nutrition Info:** Calories: 295; Fat: 8g; Protein:23g; Sugar:2g

164. Zucchini Stew

Servings: 4
Cooking Time: 12 Minutes
Ingredients:

- 8 zucchinis, roughly cubed
- ¼ cup tomato sauce
- 1 tbsp. olive oil
- ½ tsp. basil; chopped.
- ¼ tsp. rosemary; dried
- Salt and black pepper to taste.

Directions:
1. Grease a pan that fits your air fryer with the oil, add all the ingredients, toss, introduce the pan in the fryer and cook at 350°F for 12 minutes
2. Divide into bowls and serve.
- **Nutrition Info:** Calories: 200; Fat: 6g; Fiber: 2g; Carbs: 4g; Protein: 6g

165.Parmesan Chicken Meatballs

Servings: 4
Cooking Time: 12 Minutes
Ingredients:
- 1-lb. ground chicken
- 1 large egg, beaten
- ½ cup Parmesan cheese, grated
- ½ cup pork rinds, ground
- 1 teaspoon garlic powder
- 1 teaspoon paprika
- 1 teaspoon kosher salt
- ½ teaspoon pepper
- Crust:
- ½ cup pork rinds, ground

Directions:
1. Toss all the meatball Ingredients: in a bowl and mix well.
2. Make small meatballs out this mixture and roll them in the pork rinds.
3. Place the coated meatballs in the air fryer basket.
4. Press "Power Button" of Air Fry Oven and turn the dial to select the "Bake" mode.
5. Press the Time button and again turn the dial to set the cooking time to 12 minutes.
6. Now push the Temp button and rotate the dial to set the temperature at 400 degrees F.
7. Once preheated, place the air fryer basket inside and close its lid.
8. Serve warm.
- **Nutrition Info:** Calories 529 Total Fat 17 g Saturated Fat 3 g Cholesterol 65 mg Sodium 391 mg Total Carbs 55 g Fiber 6 g Sugar 8 g Protein 41g

166.Ranch Chicken Wings

Servings: 3
Cooking Time: 10 Minutes
Ingredients:
- 1/4 cup almond meal
- 1/4 cup flaxseed meal
- 2 tablespoons butter, melted
- 6 tablespoons parmesan cheese, preferably freshly grated
- 1 tablespoon Ranch seasoning mix
- 2 tablespoons oyster sauce

- 6 chicken wings, bone-in

Directions:
1. Start by preheating your Air Fryer to 370 degrees F.
2. In a resealable bag, place the almond meal, flaxseed meal, butter, parmesan, Ranch seasoning mix, andoyster sauce. Add the chicken wings and shake to coat on all sides.
3. Arrange the chicken wings in the Air Fryer basket. Spritz the chicken wings with a nonstick cooking spray.
4. Cook for 11 minutes. Turn them over and cook an additional 11 minutes. Serve warm with your favorite dipping sauce, if desired. Enjoy!
- **Nutrition Info:** 285 Calories; 22g Fat; 3g Carbs; 12g Protein; 5g Sugars; 6g Fiber

167.Turmeric Mushroom(3)

Servings: 4
Cooking Time: 12 Minutes
Ingredients:
- 1 lb. brown mushrooms
- 4 garlic cloves; minced
- ¼ tsp. cinnamon powder
- 1 tsp. olive oil
- ½ tsp. turmeric powder
- Salt and black pepper to taste.

Directions:
1. In a bowl, combine all the ingredients and toss.
2. Put the mushrooms in your air fryer's basket and cook at 370°F for 15 minutes
3. Divide the mix between plates and serve as a side dish.
- **Nutrition Info:** Calories: 208; Fat: 7g; Fiber: 3g; Carbs: 5g; Protein: 7g

168.Greek Lamb Meatballs

Servings: 12
Cooking Time: 12 Minutes
Ingredients:
- 1 pound ground lamb
- ½ cup breadcrumbs
- ¼ cup milk
- 2 egg yolks
- 1 teaspoon ground coriander
- 1 teaspoon ground cumin
- 3 garlic cloves, minced
- 1 teaspoon dried oregano
- ½ teaspoon salt
- ½ teaspoon black pepper
- 1 lemon, juiced and zested
- ¼ cup fresh parsley, chopped
- ½ cup crumbled feta cheese
- Olive oil, for shaping
- Tzatziki, for dipping

Directions:
1. Combine all ingredients except olive oil in a large mixing bowl and mix until fully incorporated.

2. Form 12 meatballs, about 2 ounces each. Use olive oil on your hands so they don't stick to the meatballs. Set aside.
3. Select the Broil function on the COSORI Air Fryer Toaster Oven, set time to 12 minutes, then press Start/Cancel to preheat.
4. Place the meatballs on the food tray, then insert the tray at top position in the preheated air fryer toaster oven. Press Start/Cancel.
5. Take out the meatballs when done and serve with a side of tzatziki.
- **Nutrition Info:** Calories: 129 kcal Total Fat: 6.4 g Saturated Fat: 0 g Cholesterol: 0 mg Sodium: 0 mg Total Carbs: 4.9 g Fiber: 0 g Sugar: 0 g Protein: 12.9 g

169.Sweet Potato Rosti

Servings: 2
Cooking Time: 15 Minutes
Ingredients:
- ½ lb. sweet potatoes, peeled, grated and squeezed
- 1 tablespoon fresh parsley, chopped finely
- Salt and ground black pepper, as required
- 2 tablespoons sour cream

Directions:
1. In a large bowl, mix together the grated sweet potato, parsley, salt, and black pepper.
2. Press "Power Button" of Air Fry Oven and turn the dial to select the "Air Fry" mode.
3. Press the Time button and again turn the dial to set the cooking time to 15 minutes.
4. Now push the Temp button and rotate the dial to set the temperature at 355 degrees F.
5. Press "Start/Pause" button to start.
6. When the unit beeps to show that it is preheated, open the lid and lightly, grease the sheet pan.
7. Arrange the sweet potato mixture into the "Sheet Pan" and shape it into an even circle.
8. Insert the "Sheet Pan" in the oven.
9. Cut the potato rosti into wedges.
10. Top with the sour cream and serve immediately.
- **Nutrition Info:** Calories: 160 Cal Total Fat: 2.7 g Saturated Fat: 1.6 g Cholesterol: 5 mg Sodium: 95 mg Total Carbs: 32.3 g Fiber: 4.7 g Sugar: 0.6 g Protein: 2.2 g

170.Chicken With Veggies And Rice

Servings: 3

Cooking Time: 20 Minutes
Ingredients:
- 3 cups cold boiled white rice
- 1 cup cooked chicken, diced
- ½ cup frozen carrots
- ½ cup frozen peas
- ½ cup onion, chopped
- 6 tablespoons soy sauce
- 1 tablespoon vegetable oil

Directions:
1. Preheat the Air fryer to 360 degree F and grease a 7" nonstick pan.
2. Mix the rice, soy sauce, and vegetable oil in a bowl.
3. Stir in the remaining ingredients and mix until well combined.
4. Transfer the rice mixture into the pan and place in the Air fryer.
5. Cook for about 20 minutes and dish out to serve immediately.
- **Nutrition Info:** Calories: 405, Fat: 6.4g, Carbohydrates: 63g, Sugar: 3.5g, Protein: 21.7g, Sodium: 1500mg

171.Chicken Caprese Sandwich

Servings: 2
Cooking Time: 3 Minutes
Ingredients:
- 2 leftover chicken breasts, or pre-cooked breaded chicken
- 1 large ripe tomato
- 4 ounces mozzarella cheese slices
- 4 slices of whole grain bread
- 1/4 cup olive oil
- 1/3 cup fresh basil leaves
- Salt and pepper to taste

Directions:
1. Start by slicing tomatoes into thin slices.
2. Layer tomatoes then cheese over two slices of bread and place on a greased baking sheet.
3. Toast in the toaster oven for about 2 minutes or until the cheese is melted.
4. Heat chicken while the cheese melts.
5. Remove from oven, sprinkle with basil, and add chicken.
6. Drizzle with oil and add salt and pepper.
7. Top with other slice of bread and serve.
- **Nutrition Info:** Calories: 808, Sodium: 847 mg, Dietary Fiber: 5.2 g, Total Fat: 43.6 g, Total Carbs: 30.7 g, Protein: 78.4 g.

DINNER RECIPES

172. Broccoli Stuffed Peppers

Servings: 2
Cooking Time: 40 Minutes
Ingredients:

- 4 eggs
- 1/2 cup cheddar cheese, grated
- 2 bell peppers, cut in half and remove seeds
  1/2 tsp garlic powder
- 1 tsp dried thyme
- 1/4 cup feta cheese, crumbled 1/2 cup broccoli, cooked
- 1/4 tsp pepper 1/2 tsp salt

Directions:

1. Preheat the air fryer to 325 F.
2. Stuff feta and broccoli into the bell peppers halved.
3. Beat egg in a bowl with seasoning and pour egg mixture into the pepper halved over feta and broccoli.
4. Place bell pepper halved into the air fryer basket and cook for 35-40 minutes.
5. Top with grated cheddar cheese and cook until cheese melted.
6. Serve and enjoy.
- **Nutrition Info:** Calories 340 Fat 22 g Carbohydrates 12 g Sugar 8.2 g Protein 22 g Cholesterol 374 mg

173. Shrimp Scampi

Servings: 6
Cooking Time: 7 Minutes
Ingredients:

- 4 tablespoons salted butter
- 1 pound shrimp, peeled and deveined
- 2 tablespoons fresh basil, chopped
- 1 tablespoon fresh chives, chopped
- 1 tablespoon fresh lemon juice
- 1 tablespoon garlic, minced
- 2 teaspoons red pepper flakes, crushed
- 2 tablespoons dry white wine

Directions:

1. Preheat the Air fryer to 325 °F and grease an Air fryer pan.
2. Heat butter, lemon juice, garlic, and red pepper flakes in a pan and return the pan to Air fryer basket.
3. Cook for about 2 minutes and stir in shrimp, basil, chives and wine.
4. Cook for about 5 minutes and dish out the mixture onto serving plates.
5. Serve hot.
- **Nutrition Info:** Calories: 250, Fat: 13.7g, Carbohydrates: 3.3g, Sugar: 0.3g, Protein: 26.3g, Sodium: 360mg

174. Herbed Eggplant

Servings: 2

Cooking Time: 15 Minutes
Ingredients:

- 1 large eggplant, cubed
- ½ teaspoon dried marjoram, crushed
- ½ teaspoon dried oregano, crushed
- ½ teaspoon dried thyme, crushed
- ½ teaspoon garlic powder
- Salt and black pepper, to taste
- Olive oil cooking spray

Directions:

1. Preheat the Air fryer to 390 degree F and grease an Air fryer basket.
2. Mix herbs, garlic powder, salt, and black pepper in a bowl.
3. Spray the eggplant cubes with cooking spray and rub with the herb mixture.
4. Arrange the eggplant cubes in the Air fryer basket and cook for about 15 minutes, flipping twice in between.
5. Dish out onto serving plates and serve hot.
- **Nutrition Info:** Calories: 62, Fat: 0.5g, Carbohydrates: 14.5g, Sugar: 7.1g, Protein: 2.4g, Sodium: 83mg

175. Couscous Stuffed Tomatoes

Servings: 4
Cooking Time: 25 Minutes
Ingredients:

- 4 tomatoes, tops and seeds removed
- 1 parsnip, peeled and finely chopped
- 1 cup mushrooms, chopped
- 1½ cups couscous
- 1 teaspoon olive oil
- 1 garlic clove, minced
- 1 tablespoon mirin sauce

Directions:

1. Preheat the Air fryer to 355 degree F and grease an Air fryer basket.
2. Heat olive oil in a skillet on low heat and add parsnips, mushrooms and garlic.
3. Cook for about 5 minutes and stir in the mirin sauce and couscous.
4. Stuff the couscous mixture into the tomatoes and arrange into the Air fryer basket.
5. Cook for about 20 minutes and dish out to serve warm.
- **Nutrition Info:** Calories: 361, Fat: 2g, Carbohydrates: 75.5g, Sugar: 5.1g, Protein: 10.4g, Sodium: 37mg

176. Easy Marinated London Broil

Servings: 4
Cooking Time: 20 Minutes
Ingredients:

- For the marinade:
- 2 tablespoons Worcestershire sauce
- 2 garlic cloves, minced

- 1 tablespoon oil
- 2 tablespoons rice vinegar
- London Broil:
- 2 pounds London broil
- 2 tablespoons tomato paste
- Sea salt and cracked black pepper, to taste
- 1 tablespoon mustard

Directions:
1. Combine all the marinade ingredients in a mixing bowl; add the London boil to the bowl. Cover and let it marinate for 3 hours.
2. Preheat the Air Fryer to 400 degrees F. Spritz the Air Fryer grill pan with cooking oil.
3. Grill the marinated London broil in the preheated Air Fryer for 18 minutes. Turn London broil over, top with the tomato paste, salt, black pepper, and mustard.
4. Continue to grill an additional 10 minutes. Serve immediately.
- **Nutrition Info:** 517 Calories; 21g Fat; 5g Carbs; 70g Protein; 4g Sugars; 7g Fiber

177.Adobe Turkey Chimichangas

Servings: 4
Cooking Time: 15 Minutes
Ingredients:
- 1 pound thickly-sliced smoked turkey from deli counter, chopped
- 1 tablespoon chili powder
- 2 cups shredded slaw cabbage
- 1 to 2 chipotles in adobo sauce
- 1 cup tomato sauce
- 3 chopped scallions
- Salt and pepper
- 4 (12-inch) flour tortillas
- 1-1/2 cups pepper jack cheese
- 2 tablespoons olive oil
- 1 cup sour cream
- 2 tablespoons chopped cilantro

Directions:
1. Start by preheating toaster oven to 400°F.
2. In a medium bowl mix together turkey and chili powder.
3. Add cabbage, chipotles, tomato sauce, and scallions; mix well.
4. Season cabbage mixture with salt and pepper and turn a few times.
5. Warm tortillas in a microwave or on a stove top.
6. Lay cheese flat in each tortilla and top with turkey mixture.
7. Fold in the top and bottom of the tortilla, then roll to close.
8. Brush baking tray with oil, then place chimichangas on tray and brush with oil.
9. Bake for 15 minutes or until tortilla is golden brown.
10. Top with sour cream and cilantro and serve.

- **Nutrition Info:** Calories: 638, Sodium: 1785 mg, Dietary Fiber: 4.2 g, Total Fat: 44.0 g, Total Carbs: 23.9 g, Protein: 38.4 g.

178.Garlic Butter Pork Chops

Servings: 4
Cooking Time: 8 Minutes
Ingredients:
- 4 pork chops
- 1 tablespoon coconut butter
- 2 teaspoons parsley
- 1 tablespoon coconut oil
- 2 teaspoons garlic, grated
- Salt and black pepper, to taste

Directions:
1. Preheat the Air fryer to 350 degree F and grease an Air fryer basket.
2. Mix all the seasonings, coconut oil, garlic, butter, and parsley in a bowl and coat the pork chops with it.
3. Cover the chops with foil and refrigerate to marinate for about 1 hour.
4. Remove the foil and arrange the chops in the Air fryer basket.
5. Cook for about 8 minutes and dish out in a bowl to serve warm.
- **Nutrition Info:** Calories: 311, Fat: 25.5g, Carbohydrates: 1.4g, Sugar: 0.3g, Protein: 18.4g, Sodium: 58mg

179.Hasselback Potatoes

Servings: 4
Cooking Time: 30 Minutes
Ingredients:
- 4 potatoes
- 2 tablespoons Parmesan cheese, shredded
- 1 tablespoon fresh chives, chopped
- 2 tablespoons olive oil

Directions:
1. Preheat the Air fryer to 355 °F and grease an Air fryer basket.
2. Cut slits along each potato about ¼-inch apart with a sharp knife, making sure slices should stay connected at the bottom.
3. Coat the potatoes with olive oil and arrange into the Air fryer basket.
4. Cook for about 30 minutes and dish out in a platter.
5. Top with chives and Parmesan cheese to serve.
- **Nutrition Info:** Calories: 218, Fat: 7.9g, Carbohydrates: 33.6g, Sugar: 2.5g, Protein: 4.6g, Sodium: 55mg

180.Steak With Cascabel-garlic Sauce

Servings: 4
Cooking Time: 20 Minutes
Ingredients:
- 2 teaspoons brown mustard

- 2 tablespoons mayonnaise
- 1 ½ pounds beef flank steak, trimmed and cubed
- 2 teaspoons minced cascabel
- ½ cup scallions, finely chopped
- 1/3 cup Crème fraîche
- 2 teaspoons cumin seeds
- 3 cloves garlic, pressed
- Pink peppercorns to taste, freshly cracked
- 1 teaspoon fine table salt
- 1/3 teaspoon black pepper, preferably freshly ground

Directions:
1. Firstly, fry the cumin seeds just about 1 minute or until they pop.
2. After that, season your beef flank steak with fine table salt, black pepper and the fried cumin seeds; arrange the seasoned beef cubes on the bottom of your baking dish that fits in the air fryer.
3. Throw in the minced cascabel, garlic, and scallions; air-fry approximately 8 minutes at 390 degrees F.
4. Once the beef cubes start to tender, add your favorite mayo, Crème fraîche, freshly cracked pink peppercorns and mustard; air-fry 7 minutes longer. Serve over hot wild rice.
- **Nutrition Info:** 329 Calories; 16g Fat; 8g Carbs; 37g Protein; 9g Sugars; 6g Fiber

181.Kale And Brussels Sprouts

Servings: 8
Cooking Time: 7 Minutes
Ingredients:
- 1 lb. Brussels sprouts, trimmed
- 3 oz. mozzarella, shredded
- 2 cups kale, torn
- 1 tbsp. olive oil
- Salt and black pepper to taste.

Directions:
1. In a pan that fits the air fryer, combine all the Ingredients: except the mozzarella and toss.
2. Put the pan in the air fryer and cook at 380°F for 15 minutes
3. Divide between plates, sprinkle the cheese on top and serve.
- **Nutrition Info:** Calories: 170; Fat: 5g; Fiber: 3g; Carbs: 4g; Protein: 7g

182.Fennel & Tomato Chicken Paillard

Servings: 1
Cooking Time: 12 Minutes
Ingredients:
- 1/4 cup olive oil
- 1 boneless skinless chicken breast
- Salt and pepper
- 1 garlic clove, thinly sliced

- 1 small diced Roma tomato
- 1/2 fennel bulb, shaved
- 1/4 cup sliced mushrooms
- 2 tablespoons sliced black olives
- 1-1/2 teaspoons capers
- 2 sprigs fresh thyme
- 1 tablespoon chopped fresh parsley

Directions:
1. Start by pounding the chicken until it is about 1/2-inch thick.
2. Preheat the toaster oven to 400°F and brush the bottom of a baking pan with olive oil.
3. Sprinkle salt and pepper on both sides of the chicken and place it in the baking pan.
4. In a bowl, mix together all other ingredients, including the remaining olive oil.
5. Spoon mixture over chicken and bake for 12 minutes.
- **Nutrition Info:** Calories: 797, Sodium: 471 mg, Dietary Fiber: 6.0 g, Total Fat: 63.7 g, Total Carbs: 16.4 g, Protein: 45.8 g.

183.Corned Beef With Carrots

Servings: 3
Cooking Time: 35 Minutes
Ingredients:
- 1 tbsp beef spice
- 1 whole onion, chopped
- 4 carrots, chopped
- 12 oz bottle beer
- 1½ cups chicken broth
- 4 pounds corned beef

Directions:
1. Preheat your air fryer to 380 f. Cover beef with beer and set aside for 20 minutes. Place carrots, onion and beef in a pot and heat over high heat. Add in broth and bring to a boil. Drain boiled meat and veggies; set aside.
2. Top with beef spice. Place the meat and veggies in your air fryer's cooking basket and cook for 30 minutes.
- **Nutrition Info:** Calories: 464 Cal Total Fat: 17 g Saturated Fat: 6.8 g Cholesterol: 91.7 mg Sodium: 1904.2 mg Total Carbs: 48.9 g Fiber: 7.2 g Sugar: 5.8 g Protein: 30.6 g

184.Cheese Zucchini Boats

Servings: 2
Cooking Time: 20 Minutes
Ingredients:
- 2 medium zucchinis
- ¼ cup full-fat ricotta cheese
- ¼ cup shredded mozzarella cheese
- ¼ cup low-carb, no-sugar-added pasta sauce.
- 2 tbsp. grated vegetarian Parmesan cheese
- 1 tbsp. avocado oil

- ¼ tsp. garlic powder.
- ½ tsp. dried parsley.
- ¼ tsp. dried oregano.

Directions:
1. Cut off 1-inch from the top and bottom of each zucchini.
2. Slice zucchini in half lengthwise and use a spoon to scoop out a bit of the inside, making room for filling. Brush with oil and spoon 2 tbsp. pasta sauce into each shell
3. Take a medium bowl, mix ricotta, mozzarella, oregano, garlic powder and parsley
4. Spoon the mixture into each zucchini shell. Place stuffed zucchini shells into the air fryer basket.
5. Adjust the temperature to 350 Degrees F and set the timer for 20 minutes
6. To remove from the fryer basket, use tongs or a spatula and carefully lift out. Top with Parmesan. Serve immediately.
- **Nutrition Info:** Calories: 215; Protein: 15g; Fiber: 7g; Fat: 19g; Carbs: 3g

185. Chat Masala Grilled Snapper

Servings: 5
Cooking Time: 25 Minutes
Ingredients:
- 2 ½ pounds whole fish
- Salt to taste
- 1/3 cup chat masala
- 3 tablespoons fresh lime juice
- 5 tablespoons olive oil

Directions:
1. Place the instant pot air fryer lid on and preheat the instant pot at 390 degrees F.
2. Place the grill pan accessory in the instant pot.
3. Season the fish with salt, chat masala and lime juice.
4. Brush with oil
5. Place the fish on a foil basket and place it inside the grill.
6. Close the air fryer lid and cook for 25 minutes.
- **Nutrition Info:** Calories:308; Carbs: 0.7g; Protein: 35.2g; Fat: 17.4g

186. Rich Meatloaf With Mustard And Peppers

Servings: 5
Cooking Time: 20 Minutes
Ingredients:
- 1 pound beef, ground
- 1/2 pound veal, ground
- 1 egg
- 4 tablespoons vegetable juice
- 1/2 cup pork rinds
- 2 bell peppers, chopped

- 1 onion, chopped
- 2 garlic cloves, minced
- 2 tablespoons tomato paste
- 2 tablespoons soy sauce
- 1 (1-ouncepackage ranch dressing mix
- Sea salt, to taste
- 1/2 teaspoon ground black pepper, to taste
- 7 ounces tomato puree
- 1 tablespoon Dijon mustard

Directions:
1. Start by preheating your Air Fryer to 330 degrees F.
2. In a mixing bowl, thoroughly combine the ground beef, veal, egg, vegetable juice, pork rinds, bell peppers, onion, garlic, tomato paste, soy sauce, ranch dressing mix, salt, and ground black pepper.
3. Mix until everything is well incorporated and press into a lightly greased meatloaf pan.
4. Cook approximately 25 minutes in the preheated Air Fryer. Whisk the tomato puree with the mustard and spread the topping over the top of your meatloaf.
5. Continue to cook 2 minutes more. Let it stand on a cooling rack for 6 minutes before slicing and serving. Enjoy!
- **Nutrition Info:** 398 Calories; 24g Fat; 9g Carbs; 32g Protein; 3g Sugars; 6g Fiber

187. Healthy Mama Meatloaf

Servings: 8
Cooking Time: 40 Minutes
Ingredients:
- 1 tablespoon olive oil
- 1 green bell pepper, diced
- 1/2 cup diced sweet onion
- 1/2 teaspoon minced garlic
- 1-lb. ground beef
- 1 cup whole wheat bread crumbs
- 2 large eggs
- 3/4 cup shredded carrot
- 3/4 cup shredded zucchini
- salt and ground black pepper to taste
- 1/4 cup ketchup, or to taste

Directions:
1. Thoroughly mix ground beef with egg, onion, garlic, crumbs, and all the ingredients in a bowl.
2. Grease a meatloaf pan with oil or butter and spread the minced beef in the pan.
3. Press "Power Button" of Air Fry Oven and turn the dial to select the "Bake" mode.
4. Press the Time button and again turn the dial to set the cooking time to 40 minutes.
5. Now push the Temp button and rotate the dial to set the temperature at 375 degrees F.
6. Once preheated, place the beef baking pan in the oven and close its lid.

7. Slice and serve.
- **Nutrition Info:** Calories: 322 Cal Total Fat: 11.8 g Saturated Fat: 2.2 g Cholesterol: 56 mg Sodium: 321 mg Total Carbs: 14.6 g Fiber: 4.4 g Sugar: 8 g Protein: 17.3 g

188.Breaded Shrimp With Lemon

Servings: 3
Cooking Time: 14 Minutes
Ingredients:
- ½ cup plain flour
- 2 egg whites
- 1 cup breadcrumbs
- 1 pound large shrimp, peeled and deveined
- Salt and ground black pepper, as required
- ¼ teaspoon lemon zest
- ¼ teaspoon cayenne pepper
- ¼ teaspoon red pepper flakes, crushed
- 2 tablespoons vegetable oil

Directions:
1. Preheat the Air fryer to 400 degree F and grease an Air fryer basket.
2. Mix flour, salt, and black pepper in a shallow bowl.
3. Whisk the egg whites in a second bowl and mix the breadcrumbs, lime zest and spices in a third bowl.
4. Coat each shrimp with the flour, dip into egg whites and finally, dredge in the breadcrumbs.
5. Drizzle the shrimp evenly with olive oil and arrange half of the coated shrimps into the Air fryer basket.
6. Cook for about 7 minutes and dish out the coated shrimps onto serving plates.
7. Repeat with the remaining mixture and serve hot.
- **Nutrition Info:** Calories: 432, Fat: 11.3g, Carbohydrates: 44.8g, Sugar: 2.5g, Protein: 37.7g, Sodium: 526mg

189.Tasty Sausage Bacon Rolls

Servings: 4
Cooking Time: 1 Hour 44 Minutes
Ingredients:
- Sausage:
- 8 bacon strips
- 8 pork sausages
- Relish:
- 8 large tomatoes
- 1 clove garlic, peeled
- 1 small onion, peeled
- 3 tbsp chopped parsley
- A pinch of salt
- A pinch of pepper
- 2 tbsp sugar
- 1 tsp smoked paprika
- 1 tbsp white wine vinegar

Directions:

1. Start with the relish; add the tomatoes, garlic, and onion in a food processor. Blitz them for 10 seconds until the mixture is pulpy. Pour the pulp into a saucepan, add the vinegar, salt, pepper, and place it over medium heat.
2. Bring to simmer for 10 minutes; add the paprika and sugar. Stir with a spoon and simmer for 10 minutes until pulpy and thick. Turn off the heat, transfer the relish to a bowl and chill it for an hour. In 30 minutes after putting the relish in the refrigerator, move on to the sausages. Wrap each sausage with a bacon strip neatly and stick in a bamboo skewer at the end of the sausage to secure the bacon ends.
3. Open the Air Fryer, place 3 to 4 wrapped sausages in the fryer basket and cook for 12 minutes at 350 F. Ensure that the bacon is golden and crispy before removing them. Repeat the cooking process for the remaining wrapped sausages. Remove the relish from the refrigerator. Serve the sausages and relish with turnip mash.
- **Nutrition Info:** 346 Calories; 11g Fat; 4g Carbs; 32g Protein; 1g Sugars; 1g Fiber

190.Party Stuffed Pork Chops

Servings: 4
Cooking Time: 40 Minutes
Ingredients:
- 8 pork chops
- ¼ tsp pepper
- 4 cups stuffing mix
- ½ tsp salt
- 2 tbsp olive oil
- 4 garlic cloves, minced
- 2 tbsp sage leaves

Directions:
1. Preheat your air fryer to 350 f. cut a hole in pork chops and fill chops with stuffing mix. In a bowl, mix sage leaves, garlic cloves, oil, salt and pepper. Cover chops with marinade and let marinate for 10 minutes. Place the chops in your air fryer's cooking basket and cook for 25 minutes. Serve and enjoy!
- **Nutrition Info:** Calories: 364 Cal Total Fat: 13 g Saturated Fat: 4 g Cholesterol: 119 mg Sodium: 349 mg Total Carbs: 19 g Fiber: 3 g Sugar: 6 g Protein: 40 g

191.Chargrilled Halibut Niçoise With Vegetables

Servings: 6
Cooking Time: 15 Minutes
Ingredients:
- 1 ½ pounds halibut fillets
- Salt and pepper to taste
- 2 tablespoons olive oil

- 2 pounds mixed vegetables
- 4 cups torn lettuce leaves
- 1 cup cherry tomatoes, halved
- 4 large hard-boiled eggs, peeled and sliced

Directions:
1. Place the instant pot air fryer lid on and preheat the instant pot at 390 degrees F.
2. Place the grill pan accessory in the instant pot.
3. Rub the halibut with salt and pepper. Brush the fish with oil.
4. Place on the grill.
5. Surround the fish fillet with the mixed vegetables, close the air fryer lid and grill for 15 minutes.
6. Assemble the salad by serving the fish fillet with mixed grilled vegetables, lettuce, cherry tomatoes, and hard-boiled eggs.
- **Nutrition Info:** Calories: 312; Carbs:16.8 g; Protein: 19.8g; Fat: 18.3g

192.Italian Shrimp Scampi

Servings: 4
Cooking Time: 20 Minutes
Ingredients:
- 2 egg whites
- 1/2 cup coconut flour
- 1 cup Parmigiano-Reggiano, grated
- 1/2 teaspoon celery seeds
- 1/2 teaspoon porcini powder
- 1/2 teaspoon onion powder
- 1 teaspoon garlic powder
- 1/2 teaspoon dried rosemary
- 1/2 teaspoon sea salt
- 1/2 teaspoon ground black pepper
- 1 ½ pounds shrimp, deveined

Directions:
1. Whisk the egg with coconut flour and Parmigiano-Reggiano. Add in seasonings and mix to combine well.
2. Dip your shrimp in the batter. Roll until they are covered on all sides.
3. Cook in the preheated Air Fryer at 390 degrees F for 5 to 7 minutes or until golden brown. Work in batches. Serve with lemon wedges if desired.
- **Nutrition Info:** 300 Calories; 13g Fat; 5g Carbs; 47g Protein; 8g Sugars; 2g Fiber

193.Amazing Bacon And Potato Platter

Servings: 4
Cooking Time: 40 Minutes
Ingredients:
- 4 potatoes, halved
- 6 garlic cloves, squashed
- 4 streaky cut rashers bacon
- 2 sprigs rosemary
- 1 tbsp olive oil

Directions:

1. Preheat your air fryer to 392 f. In a mixing bowl, mix garlic, bacon, potatoes and rosemary; toss in oil. Place the mixture in your air fryer's cooking basket and roast for 25-30 minutes. Serve and enjoy!
- **Nutrition Info:** Calories: 336 Cal Total Fat: 18.5 g Saturated Fat: 0 g Cholesterol: 82 mg Sodium: 876 mg Total Carbs: 69.9 g Fiber: 0 g Sugar: 0 g Protein: 0 g

194.Roasted Tuna On Linguine

Servings: 2
Cooking Time: 20 Minutes
Ingredients:
- 1pound fresh tuna fillets
- Salt and pepper to taste
- 1 tablespoon olive oil
- 12 ounces linguine, cooked according to package Directions:
- 2 cups parsley leaves, chopped
- 1 tablespoon capers, chopped
- Juice from 1 lemon

Directions:
1. Place the instant pot air fryer lid on and preheat the instant pot at 390 degrees F.
2. Place the grill pan accessory in the instant pot.
3. Season the tuna with salt and pepper. Brush with oil.
4. Place on the grill pan, close the air fryer lid and grill for 20 minutes.
5. Once the tuna is cooked, shred using forks and place on top of cooked linguine. Add parsley and capers. Season with salt and pepper and add lemon juice.
- **Nutrition Info:** Calories: 520; Carbs: 60.6g; Protein: 47.7g; Fat: 9.6g

195.Cheddar Pork Meatballs

Servings: 4 To 6
Cooking Time: 25 Minutes
Ingredients:
- 1 lb ground pork
- 1 large onion, chopped
- ½ tsp maple syrup
- 2 tsp mustard
- ½ cup chopped basil leaves
- Salt and black pepper to taste
- 2 tbsp. grated cheddar cheese

Directions:
1. In a mixing bowl, add the ground pork, onion, maple syrup, mustard, basil leaves, salt, pepper, and cheddar cheese; mix well. Use your hands to form bite-size balls. Place in the fryer basket and cook at 400 f for 10 minutes.
2. Slide out the fryer basket and shake it to toss the meatballs. Cook further for 5

minutes. Remove them onto a wire rack and serve with zoodles and marinara sauce.

- **Nutrition Info:** Calories: 300 Cal Total Fat: 24 g Saturated Fat: 9 g Cholesterol: 70 mg Sodium: 860 mg Total Carbs: 3 g Fiber: 0 g Sugar: 0 g Protein: 16 g

196.Award Winning Breaded Chicken

Servings: 4
Cooking Time: 20 Minutes
Ingredients:

- 1 1/2 tsp.s olive oil
- 1 tsp. red pepper flakes, crushed 1/3 tsp. chicken bouillon granules 1/3 tsp. shallot powder
- 1 1/2 tablespoons tamari soy sauce 1/3 tsp. cumin powder
- 1½ tablespoons mayo 1 tsp. kosher salt
- For the chicken:
- 2 beaten eggs Breadcrumbs
- 1½ chicken breasts, boneless and skinless 1 ½ tablespoons plain flour

Directions:

1. Margarine fly the chicken breasts, and then, marinate them for at least 55 minutes. Coat the chicken with plain flour; then, coat with the beaten eggs; finally, roll them in the breadcrumbs.
2. Lightly grease the cooking basket. Air-fry the breaded chicken at 345 °F for 12 minutes, flipping them halfway.

- **Nutrition Info:** 262 Calories; 14.9g Fat; 2.7g Carbs; 27.5g Protein; 0.3g Sugars

197.Lobster Lasagna Maine Style

Servings: 6
Cooking Time: 50 Minutes
Ingredients:

- 1/2 (15 ounces) container ricotta cheese
- 1 egg
- 1 cup shredded Cheddar cheese
- 1/2 cup shredded mozzarella cheese
- 1/2 cup grated Parmesan cheese
- 1/2 medium onion, minced
- 1-1/2 teaspoons minced garlic
- 1 tablespoon chopped fresh parsley
- 1/2 teaspoon freshly ground black pepper
- 1 (16 ounces) jar Alfredo pasta sauce
- 8 no-boil lasagna noodles
- 1 pound cooked and cubed lobster meat
- 5-ounce package baby spinach leaves

Directions:

1. Mix well half of Parmesan, half of the mozzarella, half of cheddar, egg, and ricotta cheese in a medium bowl. Stir in pepper, parsley, garlic, and onion.
2. Place the instant pot air fryer lid on, lightly grease baking pan of the instant pot with cooking spray.
3. On the bottom of the pan, spread ½ of the Alfredo sauce, top with a single layer of lasagna noodles. Followed by 1/3 of lobster meat, 1/3 of ricotta cheese mixture, 1/3 of spinach. Repeat layering process until all ingredients are used up.
4. Sprinkle remaining cheese on top. Shake pan to settle lasagna and burst bubbles. Cover pan with foil and place the baking pan in the instant pot.
5. Close the air fryer lid and cook at 360 °F for 30 minutes
6. Remove foil and cook for 10 minutes at 390 °F until tops are lightly browned.
7. Let it stand for 10 minutes.
8. Serve and enjoy.

- **Nutrition Info:** Calories: 558; Carbs: 20.4g; Protein: 36.8g; Fat: 36.5g

198.Green Beans And Mushroom Casserole

Servings: 6
Cooking Time: 12 Minutes
Ingredients:

- 24 ounces fresh green beans, trimmed
- 2 cups fresh button mushrooms, sliced
- 1/3 cup French fried onions
- 3 tablespoons olive oil
- 2 tablespoons fresh lemon juice
- 1 teaspoon ground sage
- 1 teaspoon garlic powder
- 1 teaspoon onion powder
- Salt and black pepper, to taste

Directions:

1. Preheat the Air fryer to 400 °F and grease an Air fryer basket.
2. Mix the green beans, mushrooms, oil, lemon juice, sage, and spices in a bowl and toss to coat well.
3. Arrange the green beans mixture into the Air fryer basket and cook for about 12 minutes.
4. Dish out in a serving dish and top with fried onions to serve.

- **Nutrition Info:** Calories: 65, Fat: 1.6g, Carbohydrates: 11g, Sugar: 2.4g, Protein: 3g, Sodium: 52mg

199.Beef Roast

Servings: 4
Cooking Time:x
Ingredients:

- 2 lbs. beef roast
- 1 tbsp. smoked paprika
- 3 tbsp. garlic; minced
- 3 tbsp. olive oil
- Salt and black pepper to taste

Directions:

1. In a bowl, combine all the ingredients and coat the roast well.
2. Place the roast in your air fryer and cook at 390°F for 55 minutes. Slice the roast, divide it between plates and serve with a side salad

200.Fragrant Pork Tenderloin

Servings: 3
Cooking Time: 15 Minutes
Ingredients:
- ½ teaspoon saffron
- 1 teaspoon sage
- ½ teaspoon ground cinnamon
- 1 teaspoon garlic powder
- 1 teaspoon onion powder
- 1-pound pork tenderloin
- 3 tablespoon butter
- 1 garlic clove, crushed
- 1 tablespoon apple cider vinegar

Directions:
1. Combine the saffron, sage, ground cinnamon, garlic powder, and onion powder together in the shallow bowl.
2. Then shake the spices gently to make them homogenous.
3. After this, coat the pork tenderloin in the spice mixture.
4. Rub the pork tenderloin with the crushed garlic and sprinkle the meat with the apple cider vinegar.
5. Leave the pork tenderloin for 10 minutes to marinate.
6. Meanwhile, preheat the air fryer to 320 F.
7. Put the pork tenderloin in the air fryer tray and place the butter over the meat.
8. Cook the meat for 15 minutes.
9. When the meat is cooked – let it chill briefly.
10. Slice the pork tenderloin and serve it.
11. Enjoy!
- **Nutrition Info:** calories 328, fat 16.9, fiber 0.5, carbs 2.2, protein 40

201.Herbed Carrots

Servings: 8
Cooking Time: 14 Minutes
Ingredients:
- 6 large carrots, peeled and sliced lengthwise
- 2 tablespoons olive oil
- ½ tablespoon fresh oregano, chopped
- ½ tablespoon fresh parsley, chopped
- Salt and black pepper, to taste
- 2 tablespoons olive oil, divided
- ½ cup fat-free Italian dressing
- Salt, to taste

Directions:
1. Preheat the Air fryer to 360-degree F and grease an Air fryer basket.

2. Mix the carrot slices and olive oil in a bowl and toss to coat well.
3. Arrange the carrot slices in the Air fryer basket and cook for about 12 minutes.
4. Dish out the carrot slices onto serving plates and sprinkle with herbs, salt and black pepper.
5. Transfer into the Air fryer basket and cook for 2 more minutes.
6. Dish out and serve hot.
- **Nutrition Info:** Calories: 93, Fat: 7.2g, Carbohydrates: 7.3g, Sugar: 3.8g, Protein: 0.7g, Sodium: 252mg

202.Sweet Chicken Breast

Servings: 4
Cooking Time: 12 Minutes
Ingredients:
- 1-pound chicken breast, boneless, skinless
- 3 tablespoon Stevia extract
- 1 teaspoon ground white pepper
- ½ teaspoon paprika
- 1 teaspoon cayenne pepper
- 1 teaspoon lemongrass
- 1 teaspoon lemon zest
- 1 tablespoon apple cider vinegar
- 1 tablespoon butter

Directions:
1. Sprinkle the chicken breast with the apple cider vinegar.
2. After this, rub the chicken breast with the ground white pepper, paprika, cayenne pepper, lemongrass, and lemon zest.
3. Leave the chicken breast for 5 minutes to marinate.
4. After this, rub the chicken breast with the stevia extract and leave it for 5 minutes more.
5. Preheat the air fryer to 380 F.
6. Rub the prepared chicken breast with the butter and place it in the air fryer basket tray.
7. Cook the chicken breast for 12 minutes.
8. Turn the chicken breast into another side after 6 minutes of cooking.
9. Serve the dish hot!
10. Enjoy!
- **Nutrition Info:** calories 160, fat 5.9, fiber 0.4, carbs 1, protein 24.2

203.Tasty Grilled Red Mullet

Servings: 8
Cooking Time: 15 Minutes
Ingredients:
- 8 whole red mullets, gutted and scales removed
- Salt and pepper to taste
- Juice from 1 lemon
- 1 tablespoon olive oil

Directions:
1. Place the instant pot air fryer lid on and preheat the instant pot at 390 degrees F.
2. Place the grill pan accessory in the instant pot.
3. Season the red mullet with salt, pepper, and lemon juice.
4. Place red mullets on the grill pan and brush with olive oil.
5. Close the air fryer lid and grill for 15 minutes.
- **Nutrition Info:** Calories: 152; Carbs: 0.9g; Protein: 23.1g; Fat: 6.2g

204. Pork Chops With Keto Gravy

Servings: 4
Cooking Time: 17 Minutes
Ingredients:
- 1-pound pork chops
- 1 teaspoon kosher salt
- ½ teaspoon ground cinnamon
- 1 teaspoon ground white pepper
- 1 cup heavy cream
- 6 oz. white mushrooms
- 1 tablespoon butter
- ½ teaspoon ground ginger
- 1 teaspoon ground turmeric
- 4 oz chive stems
- 1 garlic clove, chopped

Directions:
1. Sprinkle the pork chops with the kosher salt, ground cinnamon, ground white pepper, and ground turmeric.
2. Preheat the air fryer to 375 F.
3. Pour the heavy cream in the air fryer basket tray.
4. Then slice the white mushrooms and add them in the heavy cream.
5. After this, add butter, ground ginger, chopped chives, and chopped garlic.
6. Cook the gravy for 5 minutes.
7. Then stir the cream gravy and add the pork chops.
8. Cook the pork chops at 400 F for 12 minutes.
9. When the time is over stir the pork chops gently and transfer them to the serving plates.
10. Enjoy!
- **Nutrition Info:** calories 518, fat 42.4, fiber 1.5, carbs 6.2, protein 28

205. Veggie Stuffed Bell Peppers

Servings: 6
Cooking Time: 25 Minutes
Ingredients:
- 6 large bell peppers, tops and seeds removed
- 1 carrot, peeled and finely chopped
- 1 potato, peeled and finely chopped
- ½ cup fresh peas, shelled
- 1/3 cup cheddar cheese, grated
- 2 garlic cloves, minced
- Salt and black pepper, to taste

Directions:
1. Preheat the Air fryer to 350 °F and grease an Air fryer basket.
2. Mix vegetables, garlic, salt and black pepper in a bowl.
3. Stuff the vegetable mixture in each bell pepper and arrange in the Air fryer pan.
4. Cook for about 20 minutes and top with cheddar cheese.
5. Cook for about 5 more minutes and dish out to serve warm.
- **Nutrition Info:** Calories: 101, Fat: 2.5g, Carbohydrates: 17.1g, Sugar: 7.4g, Protein: 4.1g, Sodium: 51mg

206. Effortless Beef Schnitzel

Servings: 2
Cooking Time: 25 Minutes
Ingredients:
- 2 tbsp vegetable oil
- 2 oz breadcrumbs
- 1 whole egg, whisked
- 1 thin beef schnitzel, cut into strips
- 1 whole lemon

Directions:
1. Preheat your fryer to 356 F. In a bowl, add breadcrumbs and oil and stir well to get a loose mixture. Dip schnitzel in egg, then dip in breadcrumbs coat well. Place the prepared schnitzel your Air Fryer's cooking basket and cook for 12 minutes. Serve with a drizzle of lemon juice.
- **Nutrition Info:** 346 Calories; 11g Fat; 4g Carbs; 32g Protein; 1g Sugars; 1g Fiber

207. Broccoli And Tomato Sauce

Servings: 4
Cooking Time: 7 Minutes
Ingredients:
- 1 broccoli head, florets separated
- ¼ cup scallions; chopped
- ½ cup tomato sauce
- 1 tbsp. olive oil
- 1 tbsp. sweet paprika
- Salt and black pepper to taste.

Directions:
1. In a pan that fits the air fryer, combine the broccoli with the rest of the Ingredients: toss.
2. Put the pan in the fryer and cook at 380°F for 15 minutes
3. Divide between plates and serve.
- **Nutrition Info:** Calories: 163; Fat: 5g; Fiber: 2g; Carbs: 4g; Protein: 8g

208. Irish Whisky Steak

Servings: 6
Cooking Time: 20 Minutes
Ingredients:
- 2 pounds sirloin steaks

- 1 ½tablespoons tamari sauce
- 1/3 teaspoon cayenne pepper
- 1/3 teaspoon ground ginger
- 2 garlic cloves, thinly sliced
- 2 tablespoons Irish whiskey
- 2 tablespoons olive oil
- Fine sea salt, to taste

Directions:
1. Firstly, add all the ingredients, minus the olive oil and the steak, to a resealable plastic bag.
2. Throw in the steak and let it marinate for a couple of hours. After that, drizzle the sirloin steaks with 2 tablespoons olive oil.
3. Roast for approximately 22 minutesat 395 degrees F, turning it halfway through the time.
- **Nutrition Info:** 260 Calories; 17g Fat; 8g Carbs; 35g Protein; 2g Sugars; 1g Fiber

209.Crumbly Oat Meatloaf

Servings: 8
Cooking Time: 60 Minutes
Ingredients:
- 2 lbs. ground beef
- 1 cup of salsa
- 3/4 cup Quaker Oats
- 1/2 cup chopped onion
- 1 large egg, beaten
- 1 tablespoon Worcestershire sauce
- Salt and black pepper to taste

Directions:
1. Thoroughly mix ground beef with salsa, oats, onion, egg, and all the ingredients in a bowl.
2. Grease a meatloaf pan with oil or butter and spread the minced beef in the pan.
3. Press "Power Button" of Air Fry Oven and turn the dial to select the "Bake" mode.
4. Press the Time button and again turn the dial to set the cooking time to 60 minutes.
5. Now push the Temp button and rotate the dial to set the temperature at 350 degrees F.
6. Once preheated, place the beef baking pan in the oven and close its lid.
7. Slice and serve.
- **Nutrition Info:** Calories: 412 Cal Total Fat: 24.8 g Saturated Fat: 12.4 g Cholesterol: 3 mg Sodium: 132 mg Total Carbs: 43.8 g Fiber: 3.9 g Sugar: 2.5 g Protein: 18.9 g

210.Portuguese Bacalao Tapas

Servings: 4
Cooking Time: 26 Minutes
Ingredients:
- 1-pound codfish fillet, chopped
- 2 Yukon Gold potatoes, peeled and diced
- 2 tablespoon butter
- 1 yellow onion, thinly sliced
- 1 clove garlic, chopped, divided
- 1/4 cup chopped fresh parsley, divided
- 1/4 cup olive oil

- 3/4 teaspoon red pepper flakes
- freshly ground black pepper to taste
- 2 hard-cooked eggs, chopped
- 5 pitted green olives
- 5 pitted black olives

Directions:
1. Place the instant pot air fryer lid on, lightly grease baking pan of the instant pot with cooking spray. Add butter and place the baking pan in the instant pot.
2. Close the air fryer lid and melt butter at 360 °F. Stir in onions and cook for 6 minutes until caramelized.
3. Stir in black pepper, red pepper flakes, half of the parsley, garlic, olive oil, diced potatoes, and chopped fish. For 10 minutes, cook on 360 °F. Halfway through cooking time, stir well to mix.
4. Cook for 10 minutes at 390 °F until tops are lightly browned.
5. Garnish with remaining parsley, eggs, black and green olives.
6. Serve and enjoy with chips.
- **Nutrition Info:** Calories: 691; Carbs: 25.2g; Protein: 77.1g; Fat: 31.3g

211.Baked Veggie Egg Rolls

Servings: 2
Cooking Time: 20 Minutes
Ingredients:
- 1/2 tablespoon olive or vegetable oil
- 2 cups thinly-sliced chard
- 1/4 cup grated carrot
- 1/2 cup chopped pea pods
- 3 shiitake mushrooms
- 2 scallions
- 2 medium cloves garlic
- 1/2 tablespoon fresh ginger
- 1/2 tablespoon soy sauce
- 6 egg roll wrappers
- Olive oil spray for cookie sheet and egg rolls

Directions:
1. Start by mincing mushrooms, garlic, and ginger and slicing scallions.
2. Heat oil on medium heat in a medium skillet and char peas, carrots, scallions, and mushrooms.
3. Cook 3 minutes, then add ginger. Stir in soy sauce and remove from heat.
4. Preheat toaster oven to 400°F and spray cookie sheet. Spoon even portions of vegetable mix over each egg roll wrapper, and wrap them up.
5. Place egg rolls on cookie sheet and spray with olive oil. Bake for 20 minutes until egg roll shells are browned.
- **Nutrition Info:** Calories: 421, Sodium: 1166 mg, Dietary Fiber: 8.2 g, Total Fat: 7.7 g, Total Carbs: 76.9 g, Protein: 13.7 g.

212.Almond Asparagus

Servings: 3

Cooking Time: 6 Minutes
Ingredients:
- 1 pound asparagus
- 1/3 cup almonds, sliced
- 2 tablespoons olive oil
- 2 tablespoons balsamic vinegar
- Salt and black pepper, to taste

Directions:
1. Preheat the Air fryer to 400 °F and grease an Air fryer basket.
2. Mix asparagus, oil, vinegar, salt, and black pepper in a bowl and toss to coat well.
3. Arrange asparagus into the Air fryer basket and sprinkle with the almond slices.
4. Cook for about 6 minutes and dish out to serve hot.
- **Nutrition Info:** Calories: 173, Fat: 14.8g, Carbohydrates: 8.2g, Sugar: 3.3g, Protein: 5.6g, Sodium: 54mg

213.One-pan Shrimp And Chorizo Mix Grill

Servings: 4
Cooking Time: 15 Minutes
Ingredients:
- 1 ½ pounds large shrimps, peeled and deveined
- Salt and pepper to taste
- 6 links fresh chorizo sausage
- 2 bunches asparagus spears, trimmed
- Lime wedges

Directions:
1. Place the instant pot air fryer lid on and preheat the instant pot at 390 degrees F.
2. Place the grill pan accessory in the instant pot.
3. Season the shrimps with salt and pepper to taste. Set aside.
4. Place the chorizo on the grill pan and the sausage.
5. Place the asparagus on top.
6. Close the air fryer lid and grill for 15 minutes.
7. Serve with lime wedges.
- **Nutrition Info:** Calories:124 ; Carbs: 9.4g; Protein: 8.2g; Fat: 7.1g

214.Grilled Tasty Scallops

Servings: 2
Cooking Time: 10 Minutes
Ingredients:
- 1 pound sea scallops, cleaned and patted dry
- Salt and pepper to taste
- 3 dried chilies
- 2 tablespoon dried thyme
- 1 tablespoon dried oregano
- 1 tablespoon ground coriander
- 1 tablespoon ground fennel
- 2 teaspoons chipotle pepper

Directions:
1. Place the instant pot air fryer lid on and preheat the instant pot at 390 degrees F.

2. Place the grill pan accessory in the instant pot.
3. Mix all ingredients in a bowl.
4. Dump the scallops on the grill pan, close the air fryer lid and cook for 10 minutes.
- **Nutrition Info:** Calories:291 ; Carbs: 20.7g; Protein: 48.6g; Fat: 2.5g

215.Okra With Green Beans

Servings: 2
Cooking Time: 20 Minutes
Ingredients:
- ½, 10-ouncesbag frozen cut okra
- ½, 10-ouncesbag frozen cut green beans
- ¼ cup nutritional yeast
- 3 tablespoons balsamic vinegar
- Salt and black pepper, to taste

Directions:
1. Preheat the Air fryer to 400 °F and grease an Air fryer basket.
2. Mix the okra, green beans, nutritional yeast, vinegar, salt, and black pepper in a bowl and toss to coat well.
3. Arrange the okra mixture into the Air fryer basket and cook for about 20 minutes.
4. Dish out in a serving dish and serve hot.
- **Nutrition Info:** Calories: 126, Fat: 1.3g, Carbohydrates: 19.7g, Sugar: 2.1g, Protein: 11.9g, Sodium: 100mg

216.Sage Sausages Balls

Servings: 4
Cooking Time: 20 Minutes
Ingredients:
- 3 ½ oz sausages, sliced
- Salt and black pepper to taste
- 1 cup onion, chopped
- 3 tbsp breadcrumbs
- ½ tsp garlic puree
- 1 tsp sage

Directions:
1. Preheat your air fryer to 340 f. In a bowl, mix onions, sausage meat, sage, garlic puree, salt and pepper. Add breadcrumbs to a plate. Form balls using the mixture and roll them in breadcrumbs. Add onion balls in your air fryer's cooking basket and cook for 15 minutes. Serve and enjoy!
- **Nutrition Info:** Calories: 162 Cal Total Fat: 12.1 g Saturated Fat: 0 g Cholesterol: 25 mg Sodium: 324 mg Total Carbs: 7.3 g Fiber: 0 g Sugar: 0 g Protein: 6 g

217.Indian Meatballs With Lamb

Servings: 8
Cooking Time: 14 Minutes
Ingredients:
- 1 garlic clove
- 1 tablespoon butter
- 4 oz chive stems
- ¼ tablespoon turmeric
- 1/3 teaspoon cayenne pepper

- 1 teaspoon ground coriander
- ¼ teaspoon bay leaf
- 1 teaspoon salt
- 1-pound ground lamb
- 1 egg
- 1 teaspoon ground black pepper

Directions:
1. Peel the garlic clove and mince it
2. Combine the minced garlic with the ground lamb.
3. Then sprinkle the meat mixture with the turmeric, cayenne pepper, ground coriander, bay leaf, salt, and ground black pepper.
4. Beat the egg in the forcemeat.
5. Then grate the chives and add them in the lamb forcemeat too.
6. Mix it up to make the smooth mass.
7. Then preheat the air fryer to 400 F.
8. Put the butter in the air fryer basket tray and melt it.
9. Then make the meatballs from the lamb mixture and place them in the air fryer basket tray.
10. Cook the dish for 14 minutes.
11. Stir the meatballs twice during the cooking.
12. Serve the cooked meatballs immediately.
13. Enjoy!
- **Nutrition Info:** calories 134, fat 6.2, fiber 0.4, carbs 1.8, protein 16.9

218.Easy Air Fryed Roasted Asparagus

Servings: 4
Cooking Time: 10 Minutes
Ingredients:
- 1 bunch fresh asparagus
- 1 ½ tsp herbs de provence
- Fresh lemon wedge (optional)
- 1 tablespoon olive oil or cooking spray
- Salt and pepper to taste

Directions:
1. Wash asparagus and trim off hard ends
2. Drizzle asparagus with olive oil and add seasonings
3. Place asparagus in air fryer and cook on 360F for 6 to 10 minutes
4. Drizzle squeezed lemon over roasted asparagus.
- **Nutrition Info:** Calories 46 protein 2g fat 3g net carbs 1g

219.Air Fryer Buffalo Mushroom Poppers

Servings: 8
Cooking Time: 50 Minutes
Ingredients:
- 1 pound fresh whole button mushrooms
- 1/2 teaspoon kosher salt
- 3 tablespoons 1/3-less-fat cream cheese,
- 1/4 cup all-purpose flour
- Softened 1 jalapeño chile, seeded and minced
- Cooking spray

- 1/4 teaspoon black pepper
- 1 cup panko breadcrumbs
- 2 large eggs, lightly beaten
- 1/4 cup buffalo-style hot sauce
- 2 tablespoons chopped fresh chives
- 1/2 cup low-fat buttermilk
- 1/2 cup plain fat-free yogurt
- 2 ounces blue cheese, crumbled (about 1/2 cup)
- 3 tablespoons apple cider vinegar

Directions:
1. Remove stems from mushroom caps, chop stems and set caps aside. Stir together chopped mushroom stems, cream cheese, jalapeño, salt, and pepper. Stuff about 1 teaspoon of the mixture into each mushroom cap, rounding the filling to form a smooth ball.
2. Place panko in a bowl, place flour in a second bowl, and eggs in a third Coat mushrooms in flour, dip in egg mixture, and dredge in panko, pressing to adhere. Spray mushrooms well with cooking spray.
3. Place half of the mushrooms in air fryer basket, and cook for 20 minutes at 350°F. Transfer cooked mushrooms to a large bowl. Drizzle buffalo sauce over mushrooms; toss to coat then sprinkle with chives.
4. Stir buttermilk, yogurt, blue cheese, and cider vinegar in a small bowl. Serve mushroom poppers with blue cheese sauce.
- **Nutrition Info:** Calories 133 Fat 4g Saturated fat 2g Unsaturated fat 2g Protein 7g Carbohydrate 16g Fiber 1g Sugars 3g Sodium 485mg Calcium 10% DV Potassium 7% DV

220.Smoked Ham With Pears

Servings: 2
Cooking Time: 30 Minutes
Ingredients:
- 15 oz pears, halved
- 8 pound smoked ham
- 1 ½ cups brown sugar
- ¾ tbsp allspice
- 1 tbsp apple cider vinegar
- 1 tsp black pepper
- 1 tsp vanilla extract

Directions:
1. Preheat your air fryer to 330 f. In a bowl, mix pears, brown sugar, cider vinegar, vanilla extract, pepper, and allspice. Place the mixture in a frying pan and fry for 2-3 minutes. Pour the mixture over ham. Add the ham to the air fryer cooking basket and cook for 15 minutes. Serve ham with hot sauce, to enjoy!
- **Nutrition Info:** Calories: 550 Cal Total Fat: 29 g Saturated Fat: 0 g Cholesterol: 0 mg Sodium: 0 mg Total Carbs: 46 g Fiber: 0 g Sugar: 0 g Protein: 28 g

221.Filet Mignon With Chili Peanut Sauce

Servings: 4
Cooking Time: 20 Minutes
Ingredients:

- 2 pounds filet mignon, sliced into bite-sized strips
- 1 tablespoon oyster sauce
- 2 tablespoons sesame oil
- 2 tablespoons tamari sauce
- 1 tablespoon ginger-garlic paste
- 1 tablespoon mustard
- 1 teaspoon chili powder
- 1/4 cup peanut butter
- 2 tablespoons lime juice
- 1 teaspoon red pepper flakes
- 2 tablespoons water

Directions:

1. Place the beef strips, oyster sauce, sesame oil, tamari sauce, ginger-garlic paste, mustard, and chili powder in a large ceramic dish.
2. Cover and allow it to marinate for 2 hours in your refrigerator.
3. Cook in the preheated Air Fryer at 400 degrees F for 18 minutes, shaking the basket occasionally.
4. Mix the peanut butter with lime juice, red pepper flakes, and water. Spoon the sauce onto the air fried beef strips and serve warm.

- **Nutrition Info:** 420 Calories; 21g Fat; 5g Carbs; 50g Protein; 7g Sugars; 1g Fiber

222.Red Hot Chili Fish Curry

Servings: 4
Cooking Time: 20 Minutes
Ingredients:

- 2 tablespoons sunflower oil
- 1 pound fish, chopped
- 2 red chilies, chopped
- 1 tablespoon coriander powder
- 1 teaspoon red curry paste
- 1 cup coconut milk
- Salt and white pepper, to taste
- 1/2 teaspoon fenugreek seeds
- 1 shallot, minced
- 1 garlic clove, minced
- 1 ripe tomato, pureed

Directions:

1. Preheat your Air Fryer to 380 degrees F; brush the cooking basket with 1 tablespoon of sunflower oil.
2. Cook your fish for 10 minutes on both sides. Transfer to the baking pan that is previously greased with the remaining tablespoon of sunflower oil.
3. Add the remaining ingredients and reduce the heat to 350 degrees F. Continue to cook an additional 10 to 12 minutes or until everything is heated through. Enjoy!

- **Nutrition Info:** 298 Calories; 18g Fat; 4g Carbs; 23g Protein; 7g Sugars; 7g Fiber

223.Air Fryer Roasted Broccoli

Servings: 4
Cooking Time: 10 Minutes
Ingredients:

- 1 tsp. herbes de provence seasoning (optional)
- 4 cups fresh broccoli
- 1 tablespoon olive oil
- Salt and pepper to taste

Directions:

1. Drizzle or spray broccoli with olive and sprinkle seasoning throughout
2. Spray air fryer basket with cooking oil, place broccoli and cook for 5-8 minutes on 360F
3. Open air fryer and examine broccoli after 5 minutes because different fryer brands cook at different rates.

- **Nutrition Info:** Calories 61 Fat 4g protein 3g net carbs 4g

224.Greek-style Monkfish With Vegetables

Servings: 2
Cooking Time: 20 Minutes
Ingredients:

- 2 teaspoons olive oil
- 1 cup celery, sliced
- 2 bell peppers, sliced
- 1 teaspoon dried thyme
- 1/2 teaspoon dried marjoram
- 1/2 teaspoon dried rosemary
- 2 monkfish fillets
- 1 tablespoon soy sauce
- 2 tablespoons lime juice
- Coarse salt and ground black pepper, to taste
- 1 teaspoon cayenne pepper
- 1/2 cup Kalamata olives, pitted and sliced

Directions:

1. In a nonstick skillet, heat the olive oil for 1 minute. Once hot, sauté the celery and peppers until tender, about 4 minutes. Sprinkle with thyme, marjoram, and rosemary and set aside.
2. Toss the fish fillets with the soy sauce, lime juice, salt, black pepper, and cayenne pepper. Place the fish fillets in a lightly greased cooking basket and bake at 390 degrees F for 8 minutes.
3. Turn them over, add the olives, and cook an additional 4 minutes. Serve with the sautéed vegetables on the side.

- **Nutrition Info:** 292 Calories; 11g Fat; 1g Carbs; 22g Protein; 9g Sugars; 6g Fiber

225.Curried Eggplant

Servings: 2
Cooking Time: 10 Minutes
Ingredients:

- 1 large eggplant, cut into ½-inch thick slices
- 1 garlic clove, minced
- ½ fresh red chili, chopped

- 1 tablespoon vegetable oil
- ¼ teaspoon curry powder
- Salt, to taste

Directions:
1. Preheat the Air fryer to 300 degree F and grease an Air fryer basket.
2. Mix all the ingredients in a bowl and toss to coat well.
3. Arrange the eggplant slices in the Air fryer basket and cook for about 10 minutes, tossing once in between.
4. Dish out onto serving plates and serve hot.
- **Nutrition Info:** Calories: 121, Fat: 7.3g, Carbohydrates: 14.2g, Sugar: 7g, Protein: 2.4g, Sodium: 83mg

226.Grilled Halibut With Tomatoes And Hearts Of Palm

Servings: 4
Cooking Time: 15 Minutes
Ingredients:
- 4 halibut fillets
- Juice from 1 lemon
- Salt and pepper to taste
- 2 tablespoons oil
- ½ cup hearts of palm, rinse and drained
- 1 cup cherry tomatoes

Directions:
1. Place the instant pot air fryer lid on and preheat the instant pot at 390 degrees F.
2. Place the grill pan accessory in the instant pot.
3. Season the halibut fillets with lemon juice, salt, and pepper. Brush with oil.
4. Place the fish on the grill pan.
5. Arrange the hearts of palms and cherry tomatoes on the side and sprinkle with more salt and pepper.
6. Close the air fryer lid and cook for 15 minutes.
- **Nutrition Info:** Calories: 208; Carbs: 7g; Protein: 21 g; Fat: 11g

227.Bbq Pork Ribs

Servings: 2 To 3
Cooking Time: 5 Hrs 30 Minutes
Ingredients:
- 1 lb pork ribs
- 1 tsp soy sauce
- Salt and black pepper to taste

- 1 tsp oregano
- 1 tbsp + 1 tbsp maple syrup
- 3 tbsp barbecue sauce
- 2 cloves garlic, minced
- 1 tbsp cayenne pepper
- 1 tsp sesame oil

Directions:
1. Put the chops on a chopping board and use a knife to cut them into smaller pieces of desired sizes. Put them in a mixing bowl, add the soy sauce, salt, pepper, oregano, one tablespoon of maple syrup, barbecue sauce, garlic, cayenne pepper, and sesame oil. Mix well and place the pork in the fridge to marinate in the spices for 5 hours.
2. Preheat the Air Fryer to 350 F. Open the Air Fryer and place the ribs in the fryer basket. Slide the fryer basket in and cook for 15 minutes. Open the Air fryer, turn the ribs using tongs, apply the remaining maple syrup with a brush, close the Air Fryer, and continue cooking for 10 minutes.
- **Nutrition Info:** 346 Calories; 11g Fat; 4g Carbs; 32g Protein; 1g Sugars; 1g Fiber

228.Stuffed Okra

Servings: 2
Cooking Time: 12 Minutes
Ingredients:
- 8 ounces large okra
- ¼ cup chickpea flour
- ¼ of onion, chopped
- 2 tablespoons coconut, grated freshly
- 1 teaspoon garam masala powder
- ½ teaspoon ground turmeric
- ½ teaspoon red chili powder
- ½ teaspoon ground cumin
- Salt, to taste

Directions:
1. Preheat the Air fryer to 390 °F and grease an Air fryer basket.
2. Mix the flour, onion, grated coconut, and spices in a bowl and toss to coat well.
3. Stuff the flour mixture into okra and arrange into the Air fryer basket.
4. Cook for about 12 minutes and dish out in a serving plate.
- **Nutrition Info:** Calories: 166, Fat: 3.7g, Carbohydrates: 26.6g, Sugar: 5.3g, Protein: 7.6g, Sodium: 103mg

MEAT RECIPES

229.Golden Lamb Chops

Servings:4
Cooking Time: 25 Minutes
Ingredients:

- 1 cup all-purpose flour
- 2 teaspoons dried sage leaves
- 2 teaspoons garlic powder
- 1 tablespoon mild paprika
- 1 tablespoon salt
- 4 (6-ounce / 170-g) bone-in lamb shoulder chops, fat trimmed
- Cooking spray

Directions:

1. Spritz the air fryer basket with cooking spray.
2. Combine the flour, sage leaves, garlic powder, paprika, and salt in a large bowl. Stir to mix well. Dunk in the lamb chops and toss to coat well.
3. Arrange the lamb chops in the pan and spritz with cooking spray.
4. Put the air fryer basket on the baking pan and slide into Rack Position 2, select Air Fry, set temperature to 375ºF (190ºC) and set time to 25 minutes.
5. Flip the chops halfway through.
6. When cooking is complete, the chops should be golden brown and reaches your desired doneness.
7. Serve immediately.

230.Hawaiian Chicken Bites

Servings:4
Cooking Time: 15 Minutes
Ingredients:

- ½ cup pineapple juice
- 2 tablespoons apple cider vinegar
- ½ tablespoon minced ginger
- ½ cup ketchup
- 2 garlic cloves, minced
- ½ cup brown sugar
- 2 tablespoons sherry
- ½ cup soy sauce
- 4 chicken breasts, cubed
- Cooking spray

Directions:

1. Combine the pineapple juice, cider vinegar, ginger, ketchup, garlic, and sugar in a saucepan. Stir to mix well. Heat over low heat for 5 minutes or until thickened. Fold in the sherry and soy sauce.
2. Dunk the chicken cubes in the mixture. Press to submerge. Wrap the bowl in plastic and refrigerate to marinate for at least an hour.
3. Spritz the air fryer basket with cooking spray.
4. Remove the chicken cubes from the marinade. Shake the excess off and put in the basket. Spritz with cooking spray.
5. Put the air fryer basket on the baking pan and slide into Rack Position 2, select Air Fry, set temperature to 360ºF (182ºC) and set time to 15 minutes.
6. Flip the chicken cubes at least three times during the air frying.
7. When cooking is complete, the chicken cubes should be glazed and well browned.
8. Serve immediately.

231.Air Fryer Herb Pork Chops

Servings: 4
Cooking Time: 15 Minutes
Ingredients:

- 4 pork chops
- 2 tsp oregano
- 2 tsp thyme
- 2 tsp sage
- 1 tsp garlic powder
- 1 tsp paprika
- 1 tsp rosemary
- Pepper
- Salt

Directions:

1. Fit the oven with the rack in position 2.
2. Line the air fryer basket with parchment paper.
3. Mix garlic powder, paprika, rosemary, oregano, thyme, sage, pepper, and salt and rub over pork chops.
4. Place pork chops in the air fryer basket then place an air fryer basket in the baking pan.
5. Place a baking pan on the oven rack. Set to air fry at 360 F for 15 minutes.
6. Serve and enjoy.
- **Nutrition Info:** Calories 266 Fat 20.2 g Carbohydrates 2 g Sugar 0.3 g Protein 18.4 g Cholesterol 69 mg

232.Cheesy Turkey Burgers

Servings:4
Cooking Time: 25 Minutes
Ingredients:

- 2 medium yellow onions
- 1 tablespoon olive oil
- 1½ teaspoons kosher salt, divided
- 1¼ pound (567 g) ground turkey
- $^1/_3$ cup mayonnaise
- 1 tablespoon Dijon mustard
- 2 teaspoons Worcestershire sauce
- 4 slices sharp Cheddar cheese (about 4 ounces / 113 g in total)
- 4 hamburger buns, sliced

Directions:

1. Trim the onions and cut them in half through the root. Cut one of the halves in half. Grate one quarter. Place the grated onion in a large bowl. Thinly slice the remaining onions and place in a medium bowl with the oil and ½ teaspoon of kosher salt. Toss to coat. Place the onions in a single layer in the baking pan.
2. Slide the baking pan into Rack Position 2, select Roast, set temperature to 350ºF (180ºC), and set time to 10 minutes.
3. While the onions are cooking, add the turkey to the grated onion. Add the remaining kosher salt, mayonnaise, mustard, and Worcestershire sauce. Mix just until combined, being careful not to overwork the turkey. Divide the mixture into 4 patties, each about ¾-inch thick.
4. When cooking is complete, remove from the oven. Move the onions to one side of the pan and place the burgers on the pan. Poke your finger into the center of each burger to make a deep indentation.
5. Select Convection Broil, set temperature to High, and set time to 12 minutes.
6. After 6 minutes, remove the pan. Turn the burgers and stir the onions. Return the pan to the oven and continue cooking. After about 4 minutes, remove the pan and place the cheese slices on the burgers. Return the pan to the oven and continue cooking for about 1 minute, or until the cheese is melted and the center of the burgers has reached at least 165ºF (74ºC) on a meat thermometer.
7. When cooking is complete, remove from the oven. Loosely cover the burgers with foil.
8. Lay out the buns, cut-side up, on the oven rack. Select Convection Broil; set temperature to High, and set time to 3 minutes. Check the buns after 2 minutes; they should be lightly browned.
9. Remove the buns from the oven. Assemble the burgers and serve.

233.Ravioli With Beef-marinara Sauce

Servings:4
Cooking Time: 10 Minutes
Ingredients:
- 1 (20-ounce / 567-g) package frozen cheese ravioli
- 1 teaspoon kosher salt
- 1¼ cups water
- 6 ounces (170 g) cooked ground beef
- 2½ cups Marinara sauce
- ¼ cup grated Parmesan cheese, for garnish

Directions:
1. Place the ravioli in an even layer in the baking pan. Stir the salt into the water until dissolved and pour it over the ravioli.

2. Slide the baking pan into Rack Position 1, select Convection Bake, set temperature to 450ºF (235ºC), and set time to 10 minutes.
3. While the ravioli is cooking, mix the ground beef into the marinara sauce in a medium bowl.
4. After 6 minutes, remove the pan from the oven. Blot off any remaining water, or drain the ravioli and return them to the pan. Pour the meat sauce over the ravioli. Return the pan to the oven and continue cooking.
5. When cooking is complete, the ravioli should be tender and sauce heated through. Gently stir the ingredients. Serve the ravioli with the Parmesan cheese, if desired.

234.Shrimp Paste Chicken

Servings: 2
Cooking Time: 30 Minutes
Ingredients:
- 6 chicken wings
- ½ tbsp sugar
- 2 tbsp cornflour
- 1 tbsp white wine
- 1 tbsp shrimp paste
- 1 tbsp grated ginger
- ½ tbsp olive oil

Directions:
1. In a bowl, mix shrimp paste, olive oil, ginger, white wine, and sugar. Cover the chicken wings with the prepared marinade and roll in the flour.
2. Place the chicken in the greased baking dish and cook in your for 20 minutes at 350 F on Air Fry function. Serve.

235.Quail Marinade Cutlet

Servings:x
Cooking Time:x
Ingredients:
- ½ cup mint leaves
- 4 tsp. fennel
- 2 tbsp. ginger-garlic paste
- 1 small onion
- 6-7 flakes garlic (optional)
- Salt to taste
- 2 cups sliced quail
- 1 big capsicum (Cut this capsicum into big cubes)
- 1 onion (Cut it into quarters. Now separate the layers carefully.)
- 5 tbsp. gram flour
- A pinch of salt to taste
- For the filling:
- 2 cup fresh green coriander
- 3 tbsp. lemon juice

Directions:
1. You will first need to make the sauce. Add the ingredients to a blender and make a

thick paste. Slit the pieces of quail and stuff half the paste into the cavity obtained.
2. Take the remaining paste and add it to the gram flour and salt. Toss the pieces of quail in this mixture and set aside.
3. Apply a little bit of the mixture on the capsicum and onion. Place these on a stick along with the quail pieces.
4. Pre heat the oven at 290 Fahrenheit for around 5 minutes. Open the basket. Arrange the satay sticks properly. Close the basket. Keep the sticks with the quail at 180 degrees for around half an hour while the sticks with the vegetables are to be kept at the same temperature for only 7 minutes.
5. Turn the sticks in between so that one side does not get burnt and also to provide a uniform cook.

236.Tasty Turkey Meatballs

Servings: 6
Cooking Time: 25 Minutes
Ingredients:
- 2 eggs
- 2 lbs ground turkey
- 1/2 cup breadcrumbs
- 1 tsp cumin
- 1 tsp oregano
- 1/2 tsp pepper
- 1 tsp fresh mint, chopped
- 1/2 cup parsley, chopped
- 1/2 cup onion, minced
- 1 tbsp garlic, minced
- 1/2 tsp pepper
- 1 tsp salt

Directions:
1. Fit the oven with the rack in position
2. Add all ingredients into the mixing bowl and mix until well combined.
3. Make small balls from meat mixture and place onto the parchment-lined baking pan.
4. Set to bake at 375 F for 30 minutes. After 5 minutes place the baking pan in the preheated oven.
5. Serve and enjoy.
- **Nutrition Info:** Calories 362 Fat 18.7 g Carbohydrates 8.8 g Sugar 1.2 g Protein 44.9 g Cholesterol 209 mg

237.Honey & Garlic Chicken Drumsticks

Servings:4
Cooking Time: 20 Minutes
Ingredients:
- 1 lb chicken drumsticks, skin removed
- 2 tbsp olive oil
- 2 tbsp honey
- 2 garlic cloves, minced

Directions:

1. Add garlic, olive oil, and honey to a sealable zip bag. Add in chicken and toss to coat. Marinate in the fridge for 30 minutes. Add the coated chicken to the frying basket and press Start. Cook for 15 minutes at 400 F on AirFry function. Serve and enjoy!

238.Bacon Wrapped Pork Tenderloin

Servings: 4
Cooking Time: 15 Minutes
Ingredients:
- Pork:
- 1-2 tbsp. Dijon mustard
- 3-4 strips of bacon
- 1 pork tenderloin
- Apple Gravy:
- ½ - 1 tsp. Dijon mustard
- 1 tbsp. almond flour
- 2 tbsp. ghee
- 1 chopped onion
- 2-3 Granny Smith apples
- 1 C. vegetable broth

Directions:
1. Preparing the Ingredients. Spread Dijon mustard all over tenderloin and wrap the meat with strips of bacon.
2. Air Frying. Place into the air fryer oven, set temperature to 360°F, and set time to 15 minutes and cook 10-15 minutes at 360 degrees. Use a meat thermometer to check for doneness.
3. To make sauce, heat ghee in a pan and add shallots. Cook 1-2 minutes.
4. Then add apples, cooking 3-5 minutes until softened.
5. Add flour and ghee to make a roux. Add broth and mustard, stirring well to combine.
6. When the sauce starts to bubble, add 1 cup of sautéed apples, cooking till sauce thickens.
7. Once pork tenderloin I cook, allow to sit 5-10 minutes to rest before slicing.
8. Serve topped with apple gravy.
- **Nutrition Info:** CALORIES: 552; FAT: 25G; PROTEIN:29G; SUGAR:6G

239.Braised Chicken With Hot Peppers

Servings:4
Cooking Time: 27 Minutes
Ingredients:
- 4 bone-in, skin-on chicken thighs (about 1½ pounds / 680 g)
- 1½ teaspoon kosher salt, divided
- 1 link sweet Italian sausage (about 4 ounces / 113 g), whole
- 8 ounces (227 g) miniature bell peppers, halved and deseeded
- 1 small onion, thinly sliced
- 2 garlic cloves, minced

- 1 tablespoon olive oil
- 4 hot pickled cherry peppers, deseeded and quartered, along with 2 tablespoons pickling liquid from the jar
- ¼ cup chicken stock
- Cooking spray

Directions:
1. Salt the chicken thighs on both sides with 1 teaspoon of kosher salt. Spritz the baking pan with cooking spray and place the thighs skin-side down on the pan. Add the sausage.
2. Slide the baking pan into Rack Position 2, select Roast, set temperature to 375ºF (190ºC), and set time to 27 minutes.
3. While the chicken and sausage cook, place the bell peppers, onion, and garlic in a large bowl. Sprinkle with the remaining kosher salt and add the olive oil. Toss to coat.
4. After 10 minutes, remove from the oven and flip the chicken thighs and sausage. Add the pepper mixture to the pan. Return the pan to the oven and continue cooking.
5. After another 10 minutes, remove from the oven and add the pickled peppers, pickling liquid, and stock. Stir the pickled peppers into the peppers and onion. Return the pan to the oven and continue cooking.
6. When cooking is complete, the peppers and onion should be soft and the chicken should read 165ºF (74ºC) on a meat thermometer. Remove from the oven. Slice the sausage into thin pieces and stir it into the pepper mixture. Spoon the peppers over four plates. Top with a chicken thigh.

240.Chicken Thighs In Waffles

Servings:4
Cooking Time: 20 Minutes
Ingredients:
- For the chicken:
- 4 chicken thighs, skin on
- 1 cup low-fat buttermilk
- ½ cup all-purpose flour
- ½ teaspoon garlic powder
- ½ teaspoon mustard powder
- 1 teaspoon kosher salt
- ½ teaspoon freshly ground black pepper
- ¼ cup honey, for serving
- Cooking spray
- For the waffles:
- ½ cup all-purpose flour
- ½ cup whole wheat pastry flour
- 1 large egg, beaten
- 1 cup low-fat buttermilk
- 1 teaspoon baking powder
- 2 tablespoons canola oil
- ½ teaspoon kosher salt
- 1 tablespoon granulated sugar

Directions:

1. Combine the chicken thighs with buttermilk in a large bowl. Wrap the bowl in plastic and refrigerate to marinate for at least an hour.
2. Spritz the air fryer basket with cooking spray.
3. Combine the flour, mustard powder, garlic powder, salt, and black pepper in a shallow dish. Stir to mix well.
4. Remove the thighs from the buttermilk and pat dry with paper towels. Sit the bowl of buttermilk aside.
5. Dip the thighs in the flour mixture first, then into the buttermilk, and then into the flour mixture. Shake the excess off.
6. Arrange the thighs in the basket and spritz with cooking spray.
7. Put the air fryer basket on the baking pan and slide into Rack Position 2, select Air Fry, set temperature to 360ºF (182ºC) and set time to 20 minutes.
8. Flip the thighs halfway through.
9. When cooking is complete, an instant-read thermometer inserted in the thickest part of the chicken thighs should register at least 165ºF (74ºC).
10. Meanwhile, make the waffles: combine the ingredients for the waffles in a large bowl. Stir to mix well, then arrange the mixture in a waffle iron and cook until a golden and fragrant waffle forms.
11. Remove the waffles from the waffle iron and slice into 4 pieces. Remove the chicken thighs from the oven and allow to cool for 5 minutes.
12. Arrange each chicken thigh on each waffle piece and drizzle with 1 tablespoon of honey. Serve warm.

241.Mutton French Cuisine Galette

Servings:x
Cooking Time:x
Ingredients:
- 2 tbsp. garam masala
- 1 lb. minced mutton
- 3 tsp ginger finely chopped
- 1-2 tbsp. fresh coriander leaves
- 2 or 3 green chilies finely chopped
- 1 ½ tbsp. lemon juice
- Salt and pepper to taste

Directions:
1. Mix the ingredients in a clean bowl. Mold this mixture into round and flat French Cuisine Galettes. Wet the French Cuisine Galettes slightly with water.
2. Pre heat the oven at 160 degrees Fahrenheit for 5 minutes. Place the French Cuisine Galettes in the fry basket and let them cook for another 25 minutes at the same temperature. Keep rolling them over

to get a uniform cook. Serve either with mint sauce or ketchup.

242.Rustic Pork Ribs

Servings: 4
Cooking Time: 15 Minutes
Ingredients:
- 1 rack of pork ribs
- 3 tablespoons dry red wine
- 1 tablespoon soy sauce
- 1/2 teaspoon dried thyme
- 1/2 teaspoon onion powder
- 1/2 teaspoon garlic powder
- 1/2 teaspoon ground black pepper
- 1 teaspoon smoke salt
- 1 tablespoon cornstarch
- 1/2 teaspoon olive oil

Directions:
1. Preparing the Ingredients. Begin by preheating your air fryer oven to 390 degrees F. Place all ingredients in a mixing bowl and let them marinate at least 1 hour.
2. Air Frying. Cook the marinated ribs approximately 25 minutes at 390 degrees F.
3. Serve hot.

243.Mexican Salsa Chicken

Servings: 6
Cooking Time: 30 Minutes
Ingredients:
- 4 chicken breasts, skinless & boneless
- 1/4 tsp cumin
- 1/4 tsp garlic powder
- 1 3/4 cups Mexican shredded cheese
- 12 oz salsa
- 1/4 tsp pepper
- 1/4 tsp salt

Directions:
1. Fit the oven with the rack in position
2. Place chicken breasts into the baking dish and season with cumin, garlic powder, pepper, and salt.
3. Pour salsa over chicken breasts.
4. Sprinkle shredded cheese on top of chicken.
5. Set to bake at 375 F for 35 minutes. After 5 minutes place the baking dish in the preheated oven.
6. Serve and enjoy.
- **Nutrition Info:** Calories 330 Fat 17.8 g Carbohydrates 6.1 g Sugar 1.8 g Protein 36.1 g Cholesterol 116 mg

244.Teriyaki Chicken Thighs With Lemony Snow Peas

Servings:4
Cooking Time: 34 Minutes
Ingredients:
- ¼ cup chicken broth
- ½ teaspoon grated fresh ginger
- ⅛ teaspoon red pepper flakes
- 1½ tablespoons soy sauce
- 4 (5-ounce / 142-g) bone-in chicken thighs, trimmed
- 1 tablespoon mirin
- ½ teaspoon cornstarch
- 1 tablespoon sugar
- 6 ounces (170 g) snow peas, strings removed
- ⅛ teaspoon lemon zest
- 1 garlic clove, minced
- ¼ teaspoon salt
- Ground black pepper, to taste
- ½ teaspoon lemon juice

Directions:
1. Combine the broth, ginger, pepper flakes, and soy sauce in a large bowl. Stir to mix well.
2. Pierce 10 to 15 holes into the chicken skin. Put the chicken in the broth mixture and toss to coat well. Let sit for 10 minutes to marinate.
3. Transfer the marinated chicken on a plate and pat dry with paper towels.
4. Scoop 2 tablespoons of marinade in a microwave-safe bowl and combine with mirin, cornstarch, and sugar. Stir to mix well. Microwave for 1 minute or until frothy and has a thick consistency. Set aside.
5. Arrange the chicken in the air fryer basket, skin side up.
6. Put the air fryer basket on the baking pan and slide into Rack Position 2, select Air Fry, set temperature to 400ºF (205ºC) and set time to 25 minutes.
7. Flip the chicken halfway through.
8. When cooking is complete, brush the chicken skin with marinade mixture. Air fry the chicken for 5 more minutes or until glazed.
9. Remove the chicken from the oven. Allow the chicken to cool for 10 minutes.
10. Meanwhile, combine the snow peas, lemon zest, garlic, salt, and ground black pepper in a small bowl. Toss to coat well.
11. Transfer the snow peas in the basket.
12. Put the air fryer basket on the baking pan and slide into Rack Position 2, select Air Fry, set temperature to 400ºF (205ºC) and set time to 3 minutes.
13. When cooking is complete, the peas should be soft.
14. Remove the peas from the oven and toss with lemon juice.
15. Serve the chicken with lemony snow peas.

245.Chicken Wrapped In Bacon

Servings: 2
Cooking Time: 20 Minutes

Ingredients:
- 2 chicken breasts
- 8 oz onion and chive cream cheese
- 1 tbsp butter
- 6 turkey bacon
- Salt to taste
- 1 tbsp fresh parsley, chopped
- Juice from ½ lemon

Directions:
1. Preheat on Air Fry function to 390 F. Stretch out the bacon slightly and lay them in 2 sets; 3 bacon strips together on each side. Place the chicken breast on each bacon set and use a knife to smear cream cheese on both. Share the butter on top and sprinkle with salt. Wrap the bacon around the chicken and secure the ends into the wrap.
2. Place the wrapped chicken in the AirFryer basket and fit in the baking tray; cook for 14 minutes. Turn the chicken halfway through. Remove the chicken to a serving platter and top with parsley and lemon juice. Serve with steamed greens.

246. Cheesy Chicken With Tomato Sauce

Servings: 2
Cooking Time: 20 Minutes
Ingredients:
- 2 chicken breasts, ½-inch thick
- 1 egg, beaten
- ½ cup breadcrumbs
- Salt and black pepper to taste
- 2 tbsp tomato sauce
- 2 tbsp Grana Padano cheese, grated
- ¼ cup mozzarella cheese, shredded

Directions:
1. Preheat on AirFry function to 350 F. Dip the breasts into the egg, then into the crumbs and arrange on the greased basket. Cook for 5 minutes. Turn, drizzle with tomato sauce, sprinkle with Grana Padano and mozzarella cheeses, and cook for 5 more minutes. Serve warm.

247. Spicy Chicken Skewers With Satay Sauce

Servings: 4
Cooking Time: 10 Minutes
Ingredients:
- 4 (6-ounce / 170-g) boneless, skinless chicken breasts, sliced into strips
- 1 teaspoon sea salt
- 1 teaspoon paprika
- Cooking spray
- Satay Sauce:
- ¼ cup creamy almond butter
- ½ teaspoon hot sauce
- 1½ tablespoons coconut vinegar
- 2 tablespoons chicken broth

- 1 teaspoon peeled and minced fresh ginger
- 1 clove garlic, minced
- 1 teaspoon sugar
- For Serving:
- ¼ cup chopped cilantro leaves
- Red pepper flakes, to taste
- Thinly sliced red, orange, or / and yellow bell peppers
- Special Equipment:
- 16 wooden or bamboo skewers, soaked in water for 15 minutes

Directions:
1. Spritz the air fryer basket with cooking spray.
2. Run the bamboo skewers through the chicken strips, then arrange the chicken skewers in the basket and sprinkle with salt and paprika.
3. Put the air fryer basket on the baking pan and slide into Rack Position 2, select Air Fry, set temperature to 400ºF (205ºC) and set time to 10 minutes.
4. Flip the chicken skewers halfway during the cooking.
5. When cooking is complete, the chicken should be lightly browned.
6. Meanwhile, combine the ingredients for the sauce in a small bowl. Stir to mix well.
7. Transfer the cooked chicken skewers on a large plate, then top with cilantro, sliced bell peppers, red pepper flakes. Serve with the sauce or just baste the sauce over before serving.

248. Teriyaki Pork Ribs With Tomato Sauce

Servings: 3
Cooking Time: 20 Minutes + Marinating Time
Ingredients:
- 1 pound pork ribs
- Salt and black pepper to taste
- 1 tbsp sugar
- 1 tsp ginger juice
- 1 tsp five-spice powder
- 1 tbsp teriyaki sauce
- 1 tbsp soy sauce
- 1 garlic clove, minced
- 2 tbsp honey
- 1 tbsp tomato sauce
- 1 tbsp olive oil

Directions:
1. In a bowl, mix pepper, sugar, five-spice powder, salt, ginger juice, and teriyaki sauce. Add pork ribs to the marinade and let sit for 2 hours.
2. Add ribs to the greased basket and fit in the baking tray; cook for 8 minutes on Air Fry function at 350 F. In a separate bowl, mix

soy sauce, garlic, honey, 1 tbsp of water, and tomato sauce.

3. In a pan over medium heat, heat olive oil and fry garlic for 30 seconds. Add fried pork ribs and pour in the sauce. Stir-fry for a few minutes and serve.

249.Crispy Lamb Chops

Servings: 5
Cooking Time: 15 Minutes
Ingredients:
- 10 lamb chop cutlets, bone in & fat removed
- 1 cup bread crumbs
- 1 tbsp. parmesan cheese, grated
- 2 eggs
- ¼ tsp salt
- ¼ tsp pepper
- Nonstick cooking spray

Directions:
1. In a shallow dish, combine breadcrumbs and parmesan.
2. In a separate shallow dish, whisk eggs with salt and pepper.
3. Place baking pan in position 2 of the oven. Lightly spray fryer basket with cooking spray.
4. Dip chops first in egg mixture then in breadcrumbs to coat both sides. Place in single layer in the basket, these will need to be cooked in batches.
5. Place basket on the baking pan and set oven to air fry on 350°F for 6 minutes. Cook chops turning them over halfway through cooking time. Repeat with remaining chops and serve.
- **Nutrition Info:** Calories 233, Total Fat 9g, Saturated Fat 3g, Total Carbs 16g, Net Carbs 15g, Protein 22g, Sugar 1g, Fiber 1g, Sodium 386mg, Potassium 348mg, Phosphorus 240mg

250.Dijon Roasted Lamb Chops

Servings: 4
Cooking Time: 15 Minutes
Ingredients:
- 8 lamb loin chops
- 2 tbsp. Dijon mustard
- 2 tbsp. extra virgin olive oil
- 2 cloves garlic, chopped fine
- 2 tsp dried Herbs de Provence
- ¼ tsp salt
- ¼ tsp pepper

Directions:
1. Line baking pan with parchment paper.
2. Lay chops, in a single layer, on prepared pan. Sprinkle with salt and pepper.
3. In a small bowl, combine remaining ingredients, mix well. Spoon mixture over tops of chops evenly.

4. Set oven to convection bake on 400°F for 20 minutes. After 5 minutes, place pan in position 1 of the oven and cook 15 minutes.
5. Remove from oven and let rest 5 minutes before serving.
- **Nutrition Info:** Calories 189, Total Fat 13g, Saturated Fat 3g, Total Carbs 1g, Net Carbs 1g, Protein 17g, Sugar 0g, Fiber 0g, Sodium 296mg, Potassium 295mg, Phosphorus 170mg

251.Crispy Cracker Crusted Pork Chops

Servings: 3
Cooking Time: 30 Minutes
Ingredients:
- 3 pork chops, boneless
- 2 tbsp milk
- 1 egg, lightly beaten
- 1/2 cup crackers, crushed
- 4 tbsp parmesan cheese, grated
- Pepper
- Salt

Directions:
1. Fit the oven with the rack in position
2. In a shallow bowl, whisk egg and milk.
3. In a separate shallow dish, mix cheese, crackers, pepper, and salt.
4. Dip pork chops in egg then coat with cheese mixture.
5. Place coated pork chops in a baking pan.
6. Set to bake at 350 F for 35 minutes. After 5 minutes place the baking pan in the preheated oven.
7. Serve and enjoy.
- **Nutrition Info:** Calories 360 Fat 25.9 g Carbohydrates 7.2 g Sugar 0.8 g Protein 23.5 g Cholesterol 130 mg

252.Stuffed Pork Loin

Servings: 8
Cooking Time: 35 Minutes
Ingredients:
- 3 tbsp. butter
- 2 onions, sliced thin
- ½ cup beef broth
- 3 lb. pork loin, center cut
- 2 tbsp. extra virgin olive oil
- 1 tsp salt
- 1/4 tsp pepper
- 1 tsp Italian seasoning
- 2 cups gruyere cheese, grated
- Nonstick cooking spray

Directions:
1. Melt butter in a large skillet over med-high heat. Add onions and broth and cook until onions are brown and tender, about 15 minutes. Transfer to bowl and keep warm.
2. Butterfly the pork making sure you do not cut all the way through. Open up the

tenderloin, cover with plastic wrap and pound to 1/3-inch thick.

3. In a small bowl, combine salt, pepper, and Italian seasoning. Rub both sides of pork with mixture.
4. Spread half the cooked onions on one side of pork and top with half the cheese. Tightly roll up pork and tie with butcher string.
5. Heat oil in skillet. Add the tenderloin and brown on all sides.
6. Set the oven to convection bake on 425°F for 35 minutes.
7. Lightly spray the baking pan with cooking spray and place pork on it. After the oven has preheated for 5 minutes, place the baking pan in position 1 and cook 30 minutes. Basting occasionally with juice from the pan.
8. Top pork with remaining onions and cheese. Increase heat to broil and cook another 5 minutes, or until cheese is melted and golden brown. Let rest 5 minutes before slicing and serving.
- **Nutrition Info:** Calories 448, Total Fat 24g, Saturated Fat 11g, Total Carbs 3g, Net Carbs 0g, Protein 55g, Sugar 1g, Fiber 0g, Sodium 715mg, Potassium 795mg, Phosphorus 665mg

253.Sweet & Spicy Chicken

Servings: 6
Cooking Time: 30 Minutes
Ingredients:
- 6 chicken breasts, skinless, boneless, cut in 1-inch pieces
- 1 cup corn starch
- 2 cups water
- 1 cup ketchup
- ½ cup brown sugar
- 1 tbsp. sesame oil
- 3 tbsp. soy sauce
- 2 tbsp. black sesame seeds
- 2 tbsp. white sesame seeds
- ½ tsp red pepper flakes
- ½ tsp garlic powder
- 2 tbsp. green onion, chopped

Directions:
1. Place baking pan in position 2. Lightly spray fryer basket with cooking spray.
2. Place the cornstarch in a large bowl. Add chicken and toss to coat chicken thoroughly.
3. Working in batches, place chicken in a single layer in the basket and place on baking pan. Set oven to air fryer on 350°F for 10 minutes. Stir the chicken halfway through cooking time. Transfer chicken to baking sheet.
4. In a large skillet over medium heat, whisk together remaining ingredients, except

green onion. Bring to a boil, stirring occasionally. Cook until sauce has thickened, about 3-5 minutes.
5. Add chicken and stir to coat. Cook another 3-5 minutes, stirring frequently. Serve garnished with green onions.
- **Nutrition Info:** Calories 556, Total Fat 12g, Saturated Fat 3g, Total Carbs 50g, Net Carbs 49g, Protein 62g, Sugar 26g, Fiber 1g, Sodium 730mg, Potassium 957mg, Phosphorus 569mg

254.Cheesy Chicken Fritters

Servings: 17 Fritters
Cooking Time: 20 Minutes
Ingredients:
- Chicken Fritters:
- ½ tsp. salt
- 1/8 tsp. pepper
- 1 ½ tbsp. fresh dill
- 1 1/3 C. shredded mozzarella cheese
- 1/3 C. coconut flour
- 1/3 C. vegan mayo
- 2 eggs
- 1 ½ pounds chicken breasts
- Garlic Dip:
- 1/8 tsp. pepper
- ¼ tsp. salt
- ½ tbsp. lemon juice
- 1 pressed garlic cloves
- 1/3 C. vegan mayo

Directions:
1. Preparing the Ingredients. Slice chicken breasts into 1/3" pieces and place in a bowl. Add all remaining fritter ingredients to the bowl and stir well. Cover and chill 2 hours or overnight.
2. Ensure your air fryer oven is preheated to 350 degrees. Spray basket with a bit of olive oil.
3. Air Frying. Add marinated chicken to the air fryer oven. Set temperature to 350°F, and set time to 20 minutes and cook 20 minutes, making sure to turn halfway through cooking process.
4. To make the dipping sauce, combine all the dip ingredients until smooth.
- **Nutrition Info:** CALORIES: 467; FAT: 27G; PROTEIN:21G; SUGAR:3G

255.Pork Schnitzels With Sour Cream And Dill Sauce

Servings:4 To 6
Cooking Time: 4 Minutes
Ingredients:
- ½ cup flour
- 1½ teaspoons salt
- Freshly ground black pepper, to taste
- 2 eggs

- ½ cup milk
- 1½ cups toasted bread crumbs
- 1 teaspoon paprika
- 6 boneless, center cut pork chops (about 1½ pounds / 680 g), fat trimmed, pound to ½-inch thick
- 2 tablespoons olive oil
- 3 tablespoons melted butter
- Lemon wedges, for serving
- Sour Cream and Dill Sauce:
- 1 cup chicken stock
- 1½ tablespoons cornstarch
- $^1/_3$ cup sour cream
- 1½ tablespoons chopped fresh dill
- Salt and ground black pepper, to taste

Directions:

1. Combine the flour with salt and black pepper in a large bowl. Stir to mix well. Whisk the egg with milk in a second bowl. Stir the bread crumbs and paprika in a third bowl.
2. Dredge the pork chops in the flour bowl, then in the egg milk, and then into the bread crumbs bowl. Press to coat well. Shake the excess off.
3. Arrange the pork chop in the basket, then brush with olive oil and butter on all sides.
4. Put the air fryer basket on the baking pan and slide into Rack Position 2, select Air Fry, set temperature to 400ºF (205ºC) and set time to 4 minutes.
5. After 2 minutes, remove from the oven. Flip the pork. Return to the oven and continue cooking.
6. When cooking is complete, the pork chop should be golden brown and crispy.
7. Meanwhile, combine the chicken stock and cornstarch in a small saucepan and bring to a boil over medium-high heat. Simmer for 2 more minutes.
8. Turn off the heat, then mix in the sour cream, fresh dill, salt, and black pepper.
9. Remove the schnitzels from the oven to a plate and baste with sour cream and dill sauce. Squeeze the lemon wedges over and slice to serve.

256.Sriracha Beef And Broccoli

Servings:4
Cooking Time: 15 Minutes
Ingredients:
- 12 ounces (340 g) broccoli, cut into florets (about 4 cups)
- 1 pound (454 g) flat iron steak, cut into thin strips
- ½ teaspoon kosher salt
- ¾ cup soy sauce
- 1 teaspoon Sriracha sauce
- 3 tablespoons freshly squeezed orange juice

- 1 teaspoon cornstarch
- 1 medium onion, thinly sliced

Directions:

1. Line the baking pan with aluminum foil. Place the broccoli on top and sprinkle with 3 tablespoons of water. Seal the broccoli in the foil in a single layer.
2. Slide the baking pan into Rack Position 2, select Roast, set temperature to 375ºF (190ºC), and set time to 6 minutes.
3. While the broccoli steams, sprinkle the steak with the salt. In a small bowl, whisk together the soy sauce, Sriracha, orange juice, and cornstarch. Place the onion and beef in a large bowl.
4. When cooking is complete, remove from the oven. Open the packet of broccoli and use tongs to transfer the broccoli to the bowl with the beef and onion, discarding the foil and remaining water. Pour the sauce over the beef and vegetables and toss to coat. Place the mixture in the baking pan.
5. Select Roast, set temperature to 375ºF (190ºC), and set time to 9 minutes.
6. After about 4 minutes, remove from the oven and gently toss the ingredients. Return to the oven and continue cooking.
7. When cooking is complete, the sauce should be thickened, the vegetables tender, and the beef barely pink in the center. Serve warm.

257.Buffalo Chicken Tenders

Servings: 5
Cooking Time: 25 Minutes
Ingredients:
- Nonstick cooking spray
- 2/3 cup panko bread crumbs
- ½ tsp cayenne pepper
- ½ tsp paprika
- ½ tsp garlic powder
- ½ tsp salt
- 3 chicken breasts, boneless, skinless & cut in 10 strips
- ½ cup butter, melted
- ½ cup hot sauce

Directions:

1. Line a baking sheet with foil and spray with cooking spray.
2. In a shallow dish combine, bread crumbs and seasonings.
3. Dip chicken in crumb mixture to coat all sides. Lay on prepared pan and refrigerate 1 hour.
4. In a small bowl, whisk together butter and hot sauce.
5. Place baking pan in position 2 of the oven. Lightly spray the fryer basket with cooking spray.

6. Dip each piece of chicken in the butter mixture and place in basket. Place the basket on the baking pan.
7. Set oven to air fry on 400°F for 25 minutes. Cook until outside is crispy and golden brown and chicken is no longer pink. Turn chicken over halfway through cooking time. Serve immediately.
- **Nutrition Info:** Calories 371, Total Fat 23g, Saturated Fat 12g, Total Carbs 10g, Net Carbs 9g, Protein 31g, Sugar 1g, Fiber 1g, Sodium 733mg, Potassium 505mg, Phosphorus 310mg

258.Tender Baby Back Ribs

Servings: 4
Cooking Time: 45 Minutes
Ingredients:
- 1 rack baby back ribs, separated in 2-3 rib sections
- 1 tsp salt
- 1 tsp pepper
- 2 cloves garlic, crushed
- 1 bay leaf
- 3 tbsp. white wine
- 2 tbsp. olive oil
- 1 tsp lemon juice
- ¼ tsp paprika
- 1 tsp soy sauce
- 2 thyme stems
- Nonstick cooking spray

Directions:
1. In a large bowl, combine all ingredients, except ribs, and mix well.
2. Add ribs and turn to coat all sides. Let marinate at room temperature 30 minutes.
3. Lightly spray fryer basket with cooking spray. Place baking pan in position 1 of the oven.
4. Add ribs to basket, in a single layer, and place on baking pan. Set oven to air fry on 360°F for 45 minutes. Baste ribs with marinade and turn a few times while cooking. Serve immediately.
- **Nutrition Info:** Calories 772, Total Fat 52g, Saturated Fat 10g, Total Carbs 2g, Net Carbs 2g, Protein 74g, Sugar 0g, Fiber 0g, Sodium 864mg, Potassium 1255mg, Phosphorus 749mg

259.Sumptuous Beef And Pork Sausage Meatloaf

Servings:4
Cooking Time: 25 Minutes
Ingredients:
- ¾ pound (340 g) ground chuck
- 4 ounces (113 g) ground pork sausage
- 2 eggs, beaten
- 1 cup Parmesan cheese, grated
- 1 cup chopped shallot
- 3 tablespoons plain milk
- 1 tablespoon oyster sauce
- 1 tablespoon fresh parsley
- 1 teaspoon garlic paste
- 1 teaspoon chopped porcini mushrooms
- ½ teaspoon cumin powder
- Seasoned salt and crushed red pepper flakes, to taste

Directions:
1. In a large bowl, combine all the ingredients until well blended.
2. Place the meat mixture in the baking pan. Use a spatula to press the mixture to fill the pan.
3. Slide the baking pan into Rack Position 1, select Convection Bake, set temperature to 360ºF (182ºC) and set time to 25 minutes.
4. When cooking is complete, the meatloaf should be well browned.
5. Let the meatloaf rest for 5 minutes. Transfer to a serving dish and slice. Serve warm.

260.Lamb Pops

Servings:x
Cooking Time:x
Ingredients:
- 1 cup cubed lamb
- 1 ½ tsp. garlic paste
- Salt and pepper to taste
- 1 tsp. dry oregano
- 1 tsp. dry basil
- ½ cup hung curd
- 1 tsp. lemon juice
- 1 tsp. red chili flakes

Directions:
1. Add the ingredients into a separate bowl and mix them well to get a consistent mixture. Dip the lamb pieces in the above mixture and leave them aside for some time. Pre heat the oven at 180° C for around 5 minutes.
2. Place the coated lamb pieces in the fry basket and close it properly. Let them cook at the same temperature for 20 more minutes.
3. Keep turning them over in the basket so that they are cooked properly. Serve with tomato ketchup.

261.Apricot-glazed Chicken Drumsticks

Servings: 6 Drumsticks
Cooking Time: 30 Minutes
Ingredients:
- For the Glaze:
- ½ cup apricot preserves
- ½ teaspoon tamari
- ¼ teaspoon chili powder
- 2 teaspoons Dijon mustard

- For the Chicken:
- 6 chicken drumsticks
- ½ teaspoon seasoning salt
- 1 teaspoon salt
- ½ teaspoon ground black pepper
- Cooking spray
- Make the glaze:

Directions:
1. Combine the ingredients for the glaze in a saucepan, then heat over low heat for 10 minutes or until thickened.
2. Turn off the heat and sit until ready to use.
3. Make the Chicken:
4. Spritz the air fryer basket with cooking spray.
5. Combine the seasoning salt, salt, and pepper in a small bowl. Stir to mix well.
6. Place the chicken drumsticks in the basket. Spritz with cooking spray and sprinkle with the salt mixture on both sides.
7. Put the air fryer basket on the baking pan and slide into Rack Position 2, select Air Fry, set temperature to 370ºF (188ºC) and set time to 20 minutes.
8. Flip the chicken halfway through.
9. When cooking is complete, the chicken should be well browned.
10. Baste the chicken with the glaze and air fry for 2 more minutes or until the chicken tenderloin is glossy.
11. Serve immediately.

262.Chicken Skewers With Corn Salad

Servings:4
Cooking Time: 10 Minutes
Ingredients:
- 1 pound (454 g) boneless, skinless chicken breast, cut into 1½-inch chunks
- 1 green bell pepper, deseeded and cut into 1-inch pieces
- 1 red bell pepper, deseeded and cut into 1-inch pieces
- 1 large onion, cut into large chunks
- 2 tablespoons fajita seasoning
- 3 tablespoons vegetable oil, divided
- 2 teaspoons kosher salt, divided
- 2 cups corn, drained
- ¼ teaspoon granulated garlic
- 1 teaspoon freshly squeezed lime juice
- 1 tablespoon mayonnaise
- 3 tablespoons grated Parmesan cheese
- Special Equipment:
- 12 wooden skewers, soaked in water for at least 30 minutes

Directions:
1. Place the chicken, bell peppers, and onion in a large bowl. Add the fajita seasoning, 2 tablespoons of vegetable oil, and 1½ teaspoons of kosher salt. Toss to coat evenly.

2. Alternate the chicken and vegetables on the skewers, making about 12 skewers.
3. Place the corn in a medium bowl and add the remaining vegetable oil. Add the remaining kosher salt and the garlic, and toss to coat. Place the corn in an even layer in the baking pan and place the skewers on top.
4. Slide the baking pan into Rack Position 2, select Roast, set temperature to 375ºF (190ºC), and set time to 10 minutes.
5. After about 5 minutes, remove from the oven and turn the skewers. Return to the oven and continue cooking.
6. When cooking is complete, remove from the oven. Place the skewers on a platter. Put the corn back to the bowl and combine with the lime juice, mayonnaise, and Parmesan cheese. Stir to mix well. Serve the skewers with the corn.

263.Veal And Chili

Servings:x
Cooking Time:x
Ingredients:
- 1 lb. veal (Cut into Oregano Fingers)
- 2 ½ tsp. ginger-garlic paste
- 2 tsp. soya sauce
- 1-2 tbsp. honey
- ¼ tsp. Ajinomoto
- 1 tsp. red chili sauce
- ¼ tsp. salt
- ¼ tsp. red chili powder/black pepper
- A few drops of edible orange food coloring
- 2 tbsp. olive oil
- 1 ½ tsp. ginger garlic paste
- ½ tbsp. red chili sauce
- 2 tbsp. tomato ketchup
- 1-2 tsp. red chili flakes

Directions:
1. Mix all the ingredients for the marinade and put the veal Oregano Fingers inside and let it rest overnight. Mix the breadcrumbs, oregano and red chili flakes well and place the marinated Oregano Fingers on this mixture. Cover it with plastic wrap and leave it till right before you serve to cook.
2. Pre heat the oven at 160 degrees Fahrenheit for 5 minutes. Place the Oregano Fingers in the fry basket and close it. Let them cook at the same temperature for another 15 minutes or so. Toss the Oregano Fingers well so that they are cooked uniformly.

264.Sweet Pork Meatballs With Cheddar Cheese

Servings:4
Cooking Time: 25 Minutes

Ingredients:
- 1 lb ground pork
- 1 large onion, chopped
- ½ tsp maple syrup
- 2 tsp yellow mustard
- ½ cup fresh basil leaves, chopped
- Salt and black pepper to taste
- 2 tbsp Cheddar cheese, grated

Directions:
1. In a bowl, add ground pork, onion, maple syrup, mustard, basil, salt, pepper, and cheddar cheese; mix well. Form balls. Place in the frying basket. Select AirFry function, adjust the temperature to 400 F, and press Start. Cook for 10 minutes, shake, and cook for 5 minutes.

265.Beef Steak Oregano Fingers

Servings:x
Cooking Time:x
Ingredients:
- 1 lb. boneless beef steak cut into Oregano Fingers
- 2 cup dry breadcrumbs
- 4 tbsp. lemon juice
- 2 tsp. salt
- 1 tsp. pepper powder
- 1 tsp. red chili powder
- 6 tbsp. corn flour
- 4 eggs
- 2 tsp. oregano
- 2 tsp. red chili flakes
- 1 ½ tbsp. ginger-garlic paste

Directions:
1. Mix all the ingredients for the marinade and put the beef Oregano Fingers inside and let it rest overnight. Mix the breadcrumbs, oregano and red chili flakes well and place the marinated Oregano Fingers on this mixture. Cover it with plastic wrap and leave it till right before you serve to cook. Pre heat the oven at 160 degrees Fahrenheit for 5 minutes. Place the Oregano Fingers in the fry basket and close it. Let them cook at the same temperature for another 15 minutes or so. Toss the Oregano Fingers well so that they are cooked uniformly.

266.Veal Patti With Boiled Peas

Servings:x
Cooking Time:x
Ingredients:
- ½ lb. minced veal
- ½ cup breadcrumbs
- A pinch of salt to taste
- ½ cup of boiled peas
- ¼ tsp. ginger finely chopped
- 1 green chili finely chopped
- 1 tsp. lemon juice
- 1 tbsp. fresh coriander leaves. Chop them finely
- ¼ tsp. red chili powder
- ¼ tsp. cumin powder
- ¼ tsp. dried mango powder

Directions:
1. Take a container and into it pour all the masalas, onions, green chilies, peas, coriander leaves, lemon juice, and ginger and 1-2 tbsp. breadcrumbs. Add the minced veal as well. Mix all the ingredients well. Mold the mixture into round patties. Press them gently. Now roll them out carefully.
2. Pre heat the oven at 250 Fahrenheit for 5 minutes. Open the basket of the Fryer and arrange the patties in the basket. Close it carefully. Keep the fryer at 150 degrees for around 10 or 12 minutes. In between the cooking process, turn the patties over to get a uniform cook. Serve hot with mint sauce.

267.Chili Pork Chops With Tomatoes & Rice

Servings: 4
Cooking Time: 40 Minutes + Marinating Time
Ingredients:
- 4 pork chops
- 1 lime juice
- Salt and black pepper to taste
- 1 tsp garlic powder
- 1 ½ cups white rice, cooked
- 2 tbsp olive oil
- 1 can (14.5 oz) tomato sauce
- 1 onion, chopped
- 3 garlic cloves, minced
- ½ tsp oregano
- 1 tsp chipotle chili

Directions:
1. Season pork with salt, pepper, and garlic powder. In a bowl, mix onion, garlic, chipotle, oregano, and tomato sauce. Add in the pork. Let sit for 1 hour. Then remove from the mixture and place in the basket. Fit in the baking tray and cook for 25 minutes on Air Fry at 350 F. Serve with rice.

268.Chicken Wings With Chili-lime Sauce

Servings:2
Cooking Time: 25 Minutes
Ingredients:
- 10 chicken wings
- 2 tbsp hot chili sauce
- ½ tbsp lime juice
- Salt and black pepper to taste

Directions:
1. Preheat on AirFry function to 350 F. Mix lime juice and chili sauce. Toss in the

chicken wings. Transfer them to the basket and press Start. Cook for 25 minutes. Serve.

269.Pomegranate Chicken With Couscous Salad

Servings:4
Cooking Time: 20 Minutes
Ingredients:

- 3 tablespoons plus 2 teaspoons pomegranate molasses
- ½ teaspoon ground cinnamon
- 1 teaspoon minced fresh thyme
- Salt and ground black pepper, to taste
- 2 (12-ounce / 340-g) bone-in split chicken breasts, trimmed
- ¼ cup chicken broth
- ¼ cup water
- ½ cup couscous
- 1 tablespoon minced fresh parsley
- 2 ounces (57 g) cherry tomatoes, quartered
- 1 scallion, white part minced, green part sliced thin on bias
- 1 tablespoon extra-virgin olive oil
- 1 ounce (28 g) feta cheese, crumbled
- Cooking spray

Directions:

1. Spritz the air fryer basket with cooking spray.
2. Combine 3 tablespoons of pomegranate molasses, cinnamon, thyme, and ⅛ teaspoon of salt in a small bowl. Stir to mix well. Set aside.
3. Place the chicken breasts in the basket, skin side down, and spritz with cooking spray. Sprinkle with salt and ground black pepper.
4. Put the air fryer basket on the baking pan and slide into Rack Position 2, select Air Fry, set temperature to 350ºF (180ºC) and set time to 20 minutes.
5. Flip the chicken and brush with pomegranate molasses mixture halfway through.
6. Meanwhile, pour the broth and water in a pot and bring to a boil over medium-high heat. Add the couscous and sprinkle with salt. Cover and simmer for 7 minutes or until the liquid is almost absorbed.
7. Combine the remaining ingredients, except for the cheese, with cooked couscous in a large bowl. Toss to mix well. Scatter with the feta cheese.
8. When cooking is complete, remove the chicken from the oven and allow to cool for 10 minutes. Serve with vegetable and couscous salad.

270.Baked Chicken Fritters

Servings: 4
Cooking Time: 25 Minutes

Ingredients:

- 1 lb ground chicken
- 1 cup breadcrumbs
- 1 egg, lightly beaten
- 1 garlic clove, minced
- 1 1/2 cup mozzarella cheese, shredded
- 1/2 cup shallots, chopped
- 2 cups broccoli, chopped
- Pepper
- Salt

Directions:

1. Fit the oven with the rack in position
2. Add all ingredients into the bowl and mix until well combined.
3. Make small patties and place them in a parchment-lined baking pan.
4. Set to bake at 390 F for 30 minutes. After 5 minutes place the baking pan in the preheated oven.
5. Serve and enjoy.
- **Nutrition Info:** Calories 399 Fat 13 g Carbohydrates 26.5 g Sugar 2.5 g Protein 42.6 g Cholesterol 147 mg

271.Mutton Lemon Cheney

Servings:x
Cooking Time:x
Ingredients:

- 2 lb. mutton chopped
- 4 tbsp. chopped coriander
- 3 tbsp. cream
- 2 tbsp. coriander powder
- 3 onions chopped
- 2 tsp. garam masala
- 4 tbsp. fresh mint (chopped)
- 3 tbsp. chopped capsicum
- 2 tbsp. peanut flour
- 5 green chilies-roughly chopped
- 1 ½ tbsp. ginger paste
- 1 ½ tsp. garlic paste
- 1 ½ tsp. salt
- 3 tsp. lemon juice
- 3 eggs

Directions:

1. Mix the dry ingredients in a bowl. Make the mixture into a smooth paste and coat the mutton cubes with the mixture. Beat the eggs in a bowl and add a little salt to them. Dip the cubes in the egg mixture and coat them with sesame seeds and leave them in the refrigerator for an hour. Pre heat the oven at 290 Fahrenheit for around 5 minutes.
2. Place the kebabs in the basket and let them cook for another 25 minutes at the same temperature. Turn the kebabs over in between the cooking process to get a uniform cook. Serve the kebabs with mint sauce.

272.Parmesan Herb Meatballs

Servings: 6
Cooking Time: 20 Minutes
Ingredients:
- 1 lb ground beef
- 1/2 small onion, minced
- 2 garlic cloves, minced
- 1 egg, lightly beaten
- 1 1/2 tbsp fresh basil, chopped
- 1 tbsp fresh parsley, chopped
- 1/2 tbsp fresh rosemary, chopped
- 1/4 cup parmesan cheese, grated
- 1/2 cup breadcrumbs
- Pepper
- Salt

Directions:
1. Fit the oven with the rack in position
2. Add all ingredients into the mixing bowl and mix until well combined.
3. Make small balls from the meat mixture and place them into the baking pan.
4. Set to bake at 375 F for 25 minutes. After 5 minutes place the baking pan in the preheated oven.
5. Serve and enjoy.
- **Nutrition Info:** Calories 204 Fat 6.8 g Carbohydrates 7.8 g Sugar 0.9 g Protein 26.5 g Cholesterol 98 mg

273.Mango Chicken With Avocado

Servings:2
Cooking Time: 20 Minutes + Marinating Time
Ingredients:
- 2 chicken breasts, cubed
- 1 mango, cubed
- 1 avocado, pitted and sliced
- 1 chili pepper, chopped
- 5 tbsp balsamic vinegar
- 2 tbsp olive oil
- 2 garlic cloves, minced
- ¼ tsp dried oregano
- 1 tbsp fresh parsley, chopped
- ¼ tsp mustard powder

Directions:
1. In a blender, add mango, chili pepper, mustard powder, garlic, oregano, olive oil, and balsamic vinegar and pulse until smooth. Pour the liquid over chicken and let marinate for 3 hours.
2. Preheat on AirFry function to 350 F. Transfer the chicken to the basket and press Start. Cook for 14-16 minutes. Top with avocado and parsley and serve.

274.Barbecue Chicken And Coleslaw Tostadas

Servings: 4 Tostadas
Cooking Time: 10 Minutes

Ingredients:
- Coleslaw:
- ¼ cup sour cream
- ¼ small green cabbage, finely chopped
- ½ tablespoon white vinegar
- ½ teaspoon garlic powder
- ½ teaspoon salt
- ¼ teaspoon ground black pepper
- Tostadas:
- 2 cups pulled rotisserie chicken
- ½ cup barbecue sauce
- 4 corn tortillas
- ½ cup shredded Mozzarella cheese
- Cooking spray

Directions:
1. Make the Coleslaw:
2. Combine the ingredients for the coleslaw in a large bowl. Toss to mix well.
3. Refrigerate until ready to serve.
4. Make the Tostadas:
5. Spritz the air fryer basket with cooking spray.
6. Toss the chicken with barbecue sauce in a separate large bowl to combine well. Set aside.
7. Place one tortilla in the basket and spritz with cooking spray.
8. Put the air fryer basket on the baking pan and slide into Rack Position 2, select Air Fry, set temperature to 370ºF (188ºC) and set time to 10 minutes.
9. Flip the tortilla and spread the barbecue chicken and cheese over halfway through.
10. When cooking is complete, the tortilla should be browned and the cheese should be melted.
11. Serve the tostadas with coleslaw on top.

275.Citrus Carnitas

Servings:6
Cooking Time: 25 Minutes
Ingredients:
- 2½ pounds (1.1 kg) boneless country-style pork ribs, cut into 2-inch pieces
- 3 tablespoons olive brine
- 1 tablespoon minced fresh oregano leaves
- $^1/_3$ cup orange juice
- 1 teaspoon ground cumin
- 1 tablespoon minced garlic
- 1 teaspoon salt
- 1 teaspoon ground black pepper
- Cooking spray

Directions:
1. Combine all the ingredients in a large bowl. Toss to coat the pork ribs well. Wrap the bowl in plastic and refrigerate for at least an hour to marinate.
2. Spritz the air fryer basket with cooking spray.

3. Arrange the marinated pork ribs in the pan and spritz with cooking spray.
4. Put the air fryer basket on the baking pan and slide into Rack Position 2, select Air Fry, set temperature to 400ºF (205ºC) and set time to 25 minutes.
5. Flip the ribs halfway through.
6. When cooking is complete, the ribs should be well browned.
7. Serve immediately.

276. Paprika Pork Tenderloin

Servings: 6
Cooking Time: 30 Minutes
Ingredients:
- 2 lbs pork tenderloin
- For rub:
- 1 tbsp smoked paprika
- 1/2 tsp chili powder
- 1 tbsp garlic powder
- 1 tbsp onion powder
- 1/2 tsp salt

Directions:
1. Fit the oven with the rack in position
2. In a small bowl, mix all rub ingredients.
3. Coat pork tenderloin with the rub and place in baking pan.
4. Set to bake at 425 F for 35 minutes. After 5 minutes place the baking pan in the preheated oven.
5. Slice and serve.
- **Nutrition Info:** Calories 229 Fat 5.5 g Carbohydrates 2.7 g Sugar 0.9 g Protein 40.1 g Cholesterol 110 mg

277. Chicken Madeira

Servings:x
Cooking Time:x
Ingredients:
- 2 cups Madeira wine
- 2 cups beef broth
- ½ cup shredded Mozzarella cheese
- 4 boneless, skinless chicken breasts
- 1 Tbsp salt
- Salt and freshly ground black pepper, to taste
- 6 cups water
- ½ lb. asparagus, trimmed
- 2 Tbsp extra-virgin olive oil
- 2 Tbsp chopped fresh parsley

Directions:
1. Lay the chicken breasts on a cutting board, and cover each with a piece of plastic wrap. Use a mallet or a small, heavy frying pan to pound them to ¼ inch thick. Discard the plastic wrap and season with salt and pepper on both sides of the chicken.
2. Fill oven with the water, bring to a boil, and add the salt.

3. Add the asparagus and boil, uncovered, until crisp, tender, and bright green, 2 to 3 minutes. Remove immediately and set aside. Pour out the water.
4. In oven over medium heat, heat the olive oil. Cook the chicken for 4 to 5 minutes on each side. Remove and set aside.
5. Add the Madeira wine and beef broth. Bring to a boil, reduce to a simmer, and cook for 10 to 12 minutes.
6. Return the chicken to the pot, turning it to coat in the sauce.
7. Lay the asparagus and cheese on top of the chicken. Then transfer oven to the oven broiler and broil for 3 to 4 minutes. Garnish with the parsley, if using, and serve.

278. Jalapeno Basil Lamb Patties

Servings: 4
Cooking Time: 8 Minutes
Ingredients:
- 1 lb ground lamb
- 5 basil leaves, minced
- 8 mint leaves, minced
- 1/4 cup fresh parsley, chopped
- 1 tsp dried oregano
- 1 cup goat cheese, crumbled
- 1 tbsp garlic, minced
- 1 jalapeno pepper, minced
- 1/4 tsp pepper
- 1/2 tsp kosher salt

Directions:
1. Fit the oven with the rack in position
2. Add all ingredients into the mixing bowl and mix until well combined.
3. Make the equal shape of patties from the meat mixture and place it into the baking pan.
4. Set to bake at 450 F for 13 minutes. After 5 minutes place the baking pan in the preheated oven.
5. Serve and enjoy.
- **Nutrition Info:** Calories 296 Fat 13.9 g Carbohydrates 3.7 g Sugar 0.5 g Protein 37.5 g Cholesterol 118 mg

279. Pork Grandma's Easy To Cook Wontons

Servings:x
Cooking Time:x
Ingredients:
- 1 ½ cup all-purpose flour
- ½ tsp. salt
- 2 tsp. soya sauce
- 2 tbsp. oil
- 2 tsp. ginger-garlic paste
- 2 tsp. vinegar
- 5 tbsp. water
- 2 cups minced pork

Directions:

1. Squeeze the dough and cover it with plastic wrap and set aside. Next, cook the ingredients for the filling and try to ensure that the pork is covered well with the sauce. Roll the dough and place the filling in the center.
2. Now, wrap the dough to cover the filling and pinch the edges together. Pre heat the oven at 200° F for 5 minutes. Place the wontons in the fry basket and close it.
3. Let them cook at the same temperature for another 20 minutes. Recommended sides are chili sauce or ketchup.

280.Dijon Pork Tenderloin

Servings:4
Cooking Time: 15 Minutes
Ingredients:

- 3 tablespoons Dijon mustard
- 3 tablespoons honey
- 1 teaspoon dried rosemary
- 1 tablespoon olive oil
- 1 pound (454 g) pork tenderloin, rinsed and drained
- Salt and freshly ground black pepper, to taste

Directions:

1. In a small bowl, combine the Dijon mustard, honey, and rosemary. Stir to combine.
2. Rub the pork tenderloin with salt and pepper on all sides on a clean work surface.
3. Heat the olive oil in an oven-safe skillet over high heat. Sear the pork loin on all sides in the skillet for 6 minutes or until golden brown. Flip the pork halfway through.
4. Remove from the heat and spread honey-mustard mixture evenly to coat the pork loin.
5. Select Bake of the oven, set temperature to 425ºF (220ºC) and set time to 15 minutes.
6. When cooking is complete, an instant-read thermometer inserted in the pork should register at least 145ºF (63ºC).
7. Remove from the oven and allow to rest for 3 minutes. Slice the pork into ½-inch slices and serve.

281.Strawberry-glazed Turkey

Servings:2
Cooking Time: 37 Minutes
Ingredients:

- 2 pounds (907 g) turkey breast
- 1 tablespoon olive oil
- Salt and ground black pepper, to taste
- 1 cup fresh strawberries

Directions:

1. Rub the turkey bread with olive oil on a clean work surface, then sprinkle with salt and ground black pepper.

2. Transfer the turkey in the air fryer basket and spritz with cooking spray.
3. Put the air fryer basket on the baking pan and slide into Rack Position 2, select Air Fry, set temperature to 375ºF (190ºC) and set time to 30 minutes.
4. Flip the turkey breast halfway through.
5. Meanwhile, put the strawberries in a food processor and pulse until smooth.
6. When cooking is complete, spread the puréed strawberries over the turkey and fry for 7 more minutes.
7. Serve immediately.

282.Reuben Beef Rolls With Thousand Island Sauce

Servings: 10 Rolls
Cooking Time: 10 Minutes
Ingredients:

- ½ pound (227 g) cooked corned beef, chopped
- ½ cup drained and chopped sauerkraut
- 1 (8-ounce / 227-g) package cream cheese, softened
- ½ cup shredded Swiss cheese
- 20 slices prosciutto
- Cooking spray
- Thousand Island Sauce:
- ¼ cup chopped dill pickles
- ¼ cup tomato sauce
- ¾ cup mayonnaise
- Fresh thyme leaves, for garnish
- 2 tablespoons sugar
- ⅛ teaspoon fine sea salt
- Ground black pepper, to taste

Directions:

1. Spritz the air fryer basket with cooking spray.
2. Combine the beef, sauerkraut, cream cheese, and Swiss cheese in a large bowl. Stir to mix well.
3. Unroll a slice of prosciutto on a clean work surface, then top with another slice of prosciutto crosswise. Scoop up 4 tablespoons of the beef mixture in the center.
4. Fold the top slice sides over the filling as the ends of the roll, then roll up the long sides of the bottom prosciutto and make it into a roll shape. Overlap the sides by about 1 inch. Repeat with remaining filling and prosciutto.
5. Arrange the rolls in the prepared pan, seam side down, and spritz with cooking spray.
6. Put the air fryer basket on the baking pan and slide into Rack Position 2, select Air Fry, set temperature to 400ºF (205ºC) and set time to 10 minutes.
7. Flip the rolls halfway through.

8. When cooking is complete, the rolls should be golden and crispy.
9. Meanwhile, combine the ingredients for the sauce in a small bowl. Stir to mix well.
10. Serve the rolls with the dipping sauce.

283.Easy Ranch Pork Chops

Servings: 6
Cooking Time: 35 Minutes
Ingredients:
- 6 pork chops, boneless
- 2 tbsp olive oil
- 1 oz ranch seasoning

Directions:
1. Fit the oven with the rack in position
2. Brush pork chops with oil and rub with ranch seasoning.
3. Place pork chops in a baking pan.
4. Set to bake at 400 F for 40 minutes. After 5 minutes place the baking pan in the preheated oven.
5. Serve and enjoy.
- **Nutrition Info:** Calories 311 Fat 24.6 g Carbohydrates 0 g Sugar 0 g Protein 18 g Cholesterol 69 mg

284.Turkey Burger Cutlets

Servings:x
Cooking Time:x
Ingredients:
- ½ lb. minced turkey
- ½ cup breadcrumbs
- A pinch of salt to taste
- ¼ tsp. ginger finely chopped
- 1 green chili finely chopped
- 1 tsp. lemon juice
- 1 tbsp. fresh coriander leaves. Chop them finely
- ¼ tsp. red chili powder
- ½ cup of boiled peas
- ¼ tsp. cumin powder
- ¼ tsp. dried mango powder

Directions:
1. Take a container and into it pour all the masalas, onions, green chilies, peas, coriander leaves, lemon juice, ginger and 1-2 tbsp. breadcrumbs. Add the minced turkey as well. Mix all the ingredients well.

Mold the mixture into round Cutlets. Press them gently. Now roll them out carefully. Pre heat the oven at 250 Fahrenheit for 5 minutes.
2. Open the basket of the Fryer and arrange the Cutlets in the basket. Close it carefully.
3. Keep the fryer at 150 degrees for around 10 or 12 minutes. In between the cooking process, turn the Cutlets over to get a uniform cook. Serve hot with mint sauce.

285.Air Fryer Sweet And Sour Pork

Servings: 6
Cooking Time: 12 Minutes
Ingredients:
- 3 tbsp. olive oil
- 1/16 tsp. Chinese Five Spice
- ¼ tsp. pepper
- ½ tsp. sea salt
- 1 tsp. pure sesame oil
- 2 eggs
- 1 C. almond flour
- 2 pounds pork, sliced into chunks
- Sweet and Sour Sauce:
- ¼ tsp. sea salt
- ½ tsp. garlic powder
- 1 tbsp. low-sodium soy sauce
- ½ C. rice vinegar
- 5 tbsp. tomato paste
- 1/8 tsp. water
- ½ C. sweetener of choice

Directions:
1. Preparing the Ingredients. To make the dipping sauce, whisk all sauce ingredients together over medium heat, stirring 5 minutes. Simmer uncovered 5 minutes till thickened.
2. Meanwhile, combine almond flour, five spice, pepper, and salt.
3. In another bowl, mix eggs with sesame oil.
4. Dredge pork in flour mixture and then in egg mixture. Shake any excess off before adding to air fryer rack/basket.
5. Air Frying. Set temperature to 340°F, and set time to 12 minutes.
6. Serve with sweet and sour dipping sauce!
- **Nutrition Info:** CALORIES: 371; FAT: 17G; PROTEIN:27G; SUGAR:1G

FISH & SEAFOOD RECIPES

286. Seafood Platter

Servings: x
Cooking Time: x
Ingredients:

- 1 large plate with assorted prepared seafood
- 3 tbsp. vinegar or lemon juice
- 2 or 3 tsp. paprika
- 1 tsp. black pepper
- 1 tsp. salt
- 3 tsp. ginger-garlic paste
- 1 cup yogurt
- 4 tsp. tandoori masala
- 2 tbsp. dry fenugreek leaves
- 1 tsp. black salt
- 1 tsp. chat masala
- 1 tsp. garam masala powder
- 1 tsp. red chili powder
- 1 tsp. salt
- 3 drops of red color

Directions:

1. Make the first marinade and soak the seafood in it for four hours. While this is happening, make the second marinade and soak the seafood in it overnight to let the flavors blend.
2. Pre heat the oven at 160 degrees Fahrenheit for 5 minutes. Place the Oregano Fingers in the fry basket and close it. Let them cook at the same temperature for another 15 minutes or so. Toss the Oregano Fingers well so that they are cooked uniformly. Serve them with mint sauce.

287. Piri-piri King Prawns

Servings: 2
Cooking Time: 8 Minutes
Ingredients:

- 12 king prawns, rinsed
- 1 tablespoon coconut oil
- Salt and ground black pepper, to taste
- 1 teaspoon onion powder
- 1 teaspoon garlic paste
- 1 teaspoon curry powder
- ½ teaspoon piri piri powder
- ½ teaspoon cumin powder

Directions:

1. Combine all the ingredients in a large bowl and toss until the prawns are completely coated. Place the prawns in the air fryer basket.
2. Put the air fryer basket on the baking pan and slide into Rack Position 2, select Air Fry, set temperature to 360ºF (182ºC), and set time to 8 minutes.
3. Flip the prawns halfway through the cooking time.
4. When cooking is complete, the prawns will turn pink. Remove from the oven and serve hot.

288. Crispy Coated Scallops

Servings: 4
Cooking Time: 10 Minutes
Ingredients:

- Nonstick cooking spray
- 1 lb. sea scallops, patted dry
- 1 teaspoon onion powder
- ½ tsp pepper
- 1 egg
- 1 tbsp. water
- ¼ cup Italian bread crumbs
- Paprika
- 1 tbsp. fresh lemon juice

Directions:

1. Lightly spray fryer basket with cooking spray. Place baking pan in position 2 of the oven.
2. Sprinkle scallops with onion powder and pepper.
3. In a shallow dish, whisk together egg and water.
4. Place bread crumbs in a separate shallow dish.
5. Dip scallops in egg then bread crumbs coating them lightly. Place in fryer basket and lightly spray with cooking spray. Sprinkle with paprika.
6. Place the basket on the baking pan and set oven to air fryer on 400°F. Bake 10-12 minutes until scallops are firm on the inside and golden brown on the outside. Drizzle with lemon juice and serve.

- **Nutrition Info:** Calories 122, Total Fat 2g, Saturated Fat 1g, Total Carbs 10g, Net Carbs 9g, Protein 16g, Sugar 1g, Fiber 1g, Sodium 563mg, Potassium 282mg, Phosphorus 420mg

289. Old Bay Tilapia Fillets

Servings: 4
Cooking Time: 15 Minutes
Ingredients:

- 1 pound tilapia fillets
- 1 tbsp old bay seasoning
- 2 tbsp canola oil
- 2 tbsp lemon pepper
- Salt to taste
- 2-3 butter buds

Directions:

1. Preheat your oven to 400 F on Bake function. Drizzle tilapia fillets with canola oil. In a bowl, mix salt, lemon pepper, butter

buds, and seasoning; spread on the fish. Place the fillet on the basket and fit in the baking tray. Cook for 10 minutes, flipping once until tender and crispy.

290.Parmesan Tilapia Fillets

Servings:4
Cooking Time: 15 Minutes
Ingredients:
- ¾ cup Parmesan cheese, grated
- 1 tbsp olive oil
- 1 tsp paprika
- 1 tbsp fresh parsley, chopped
- ¼ tsp garlic powder
- ¼ tsp salt
- 4 tilapia fillets

Directions:
1. Preheat on AirFry function to 350 F. In a bowl, mix parsley, Parmesan cheese, garlic, salt, and paprika. Coat in the tilapia fillets and place them in a lined baking sheet. Drizzle with the olive oil press Start. Cook cook for 8-10 minutes until golden. Serve warm.

291.Delicious Baked Basa

Servings: 4
Cooking Time: 10 Minutes
Ingredients:
- 4 basa fish fillets
- 1/4 cup green onion, sliced
- 1/2 tsp garlic powder
- 1/4 tsp lemon pepper seasoning
- 4 tbsp fresh lemon juice
- 8 tsp butter, melted
- Salt

Directions:
1. Fit the oven with the rack in position
2. Place fish fillets into the baking dish.
3. Pour remaining ingredients over fish fillets.
4. Set to bake at 425 F for 15 minutes. After 5 minutes place the baking dish in the preheated oven.
5. Serve and enjoy.
- **Nutrition Info:** Calories 214 Fat 15.3 g Carbohydrates 3.8 g Sugar 2.3 g Protein 15.4 g Cholesterol 20 mg

292.Shrimp With Smoked Paprika & Cayenne Pepper

Servings: 3
Cooking Time: 10 Minutes
Ingredients:
- 6 oz tiger shrimp, 12 to 16 pieces
- 1 tbsp olive oil
- ½ a tbsp old bay seasoning
- ¼ a tbsp cayenne pepper
- ¼ a tbsp smoked paprika
- A pinch of sea salt

Directions:
1. Preheat on Air Fry function to 380 F. Mix olive oil, old bay seasoning, cayenne pepper, smoked paprika, and sea salt in a large bowl. Add in the shrimp and toss to coat. Place the shrimp in the frying basket and fit in the baking tray; cook for 6-7 minutes, sahing once. Serve.

293.Sweet & Spicy Lime Salmon

Servings: 6
Cooking Time: 15 Minutes
Ingredients:
- 1 1/2 lbs salmon fillets
- 3 tbsp brown sugar
- 2 tbsp fresh lime juice
- 1/3 cup olive oil
- 1/2 tsp red pepper flakes
- 2 garlic cloves, minced
- Pepper
- Salt

Directions:
1. Fit the oven with the rack in position
2. Place salmon on a prepared baking sheet and season with pepper and salt.
3. In a small bowl, whisk oil, red pepper flakes, garlic, brown sugar, and lime juice.
4. Pour oil mixture over salmon.
5. Set to bake at 350 F for 20 minutes. After 5 minutes place the baking dish in the preheated oven.
6. Serve and enjoy.
- **Nutrition Info:** Calories 269 Fat 18.3 g Carbohydrates 6.1 g Sugar 4.7 g Protein 22.2 g Cholesterol 50 mg

294.Paprika Cod

Servings: 4
Cooking Time: 15 Minutes
Ingredients:
- 4 cod fillets
- 1 tsp smoked paprika
- 1/2 cup parmesan cheese, grated
- 1/2 tbsp olive oil
- 1 tsp parsley
- Pepper
- Salt

Directions:
1. Fit the oven with the rack in position
2. Brush fish fillets with oil and season with pepper and salt.
3. In a shallow dish, mix parmesan cheese, paprika, and parsley.
4. Coat fish fillets with cheese mixture and place into the baking dish.
5. Set to bake at 400 F for 20 minutes. After 5 minutes place the baking dish in the preheated oven.
6. Serve and enjoy.

- **Nutrition Info:** Calories 125 Fat 5 g Carbohydrates 0.7 g Sugar 0.1 g Protein 19.8 g Cholesterol 52 mg

295.Delicious Shrimp Casserole

Servings: 10
Cooking Time: 30 Minutes
Ingredients:
- 1 lb shrimp, peeled & tail off
- 2 tsp onion powder
- 2 tsp old bay seasoning
- 2 cups cheddar cheese, shredded
- 10.5 oz can cream of mushroom soup
- 12 oz long-grain rice
- 1 tsp salt

Directions:
1. Fit the oven with the rack in position
2. Cook rice according to the packet instructions.
3. Add shrimp into the boiling water and cook for 4 minutes or until cooked. Drain shrimp.
4. In a bowl, mix rice, shrimp, and remaining ingredients and pour into the greased 13*9-inch casserole dish.
5. Set to bake at 350 F for 35 minutes. After 5 minutes place the casserole dish in the preheated oven.
6. Serve and enjoy.
- **Nutrition Info:** Calories 286 Fat 9 g Carbohydrates 31 g Sugar 1 g Protein 18.8 g Cholesterol 120 mg

296.Baked Buttery Shrimp

Servings: 4
Cooking Time: 15 Minutes
Ingredients:
- 1 lb shrimp, peel & deveined
- 2 tsp garlic powder
- 2 tsp dry mustard
- 2 tsp cumin
- 2 tsp paprika
- 2 tsp black pepper
- 4 tsp cayenne pepper
- 1/2 cup butter, melted
- 2 tsp onion powder
- 1 tsp dried oregano
- 1 tsp dried thyme
- 3 tsp salt

Directions:
1. Fit the oven with the rack in position
2. Add shrimp, butter, and remaining ingredients into the mixing bowl and toss well.
3. Transfer shrimp mixture into the baking pan.
4. Set to bake at 400 F for 20 minutes. After 5 minutes place the baking pan in the preheated oven.
5. Serve and enjoy.

- **Nutrition Info:** Calories 372 Fat 26.2 g Carbohydrates 7.5 g Sugar 1.3 g Protein 27.6 g Cholesterol 300 mg

297.Tropical Shrimp Skewers

Servings: 4
Cooking Time: 5 Minutes
Ingredients:
- 1 tbsp. lime juice
- 1 tbsp. honey
- ¼ tsp red pepper flakes
- ¼ tsp pepper
- ¼ tsp ginger
- Nonstick cooking spray
- 1 lb. medium shrimp, peel, devein & leave tails on
- 2 cups peaches, drain & chop
- ½ green bell pepper, chopped fine
- ¼ cup scallions, chopped

Directions:
1. Soak 8 small wooden skewers in water for 15 minutes.
2. In a small bowl, whisk together lime juice, honey and spices. Transfer 2 tablespoons of the mixture to a medium bowl.
3. Place the baking pan in position 2 of the oven. Lightly spray fryer basket with cooking spray. Set oven to broil on 400°F for 10 minutes.
4. Thread 5 shrimp on each skewer and brush both sides with marinade. Place in basket and after 5 minutes, place on the baking pan. Cook 4-5 minutes or until shrimp turn pink.
5. Add peaches, bell pepper, and scallions to reserved honey mixture, mix well. Divide salsa evenly between serving plates and top with 2 skewers each. Serve immediately.
- **Nutrition Info:** Calories 181, Total Fat 1g, Saturated Fat 0g, Total Carbs 27g, Net Carbs 25g, Protein 16g, Sugar 21g, Fiber 2g, Sodium 650mg, Potassium 288mg, Phosphorus 297mg

298.Sweet Cajun Salmon

Servings: 1
Cooking Time: 10 Minutes
Ingredients:
- 1 salmon fillet
- ¼ tsp brown sugar
- Juice of ½ lemon
- 1 tbsp cajun seasoning
- 2 lemon wedges
- 1 tbsp chopped parsley

Directions:
1. Preheat on Bake function to 350 F. Combine sugar and lemon juice; coat the salmon with this mixture. Coat with the Cajun seasoning as well. Place a parchment paper on a baking tray and cook the fish in

your for 10 minutes. Serve with lemon wedges and parsley.

299.Scallops And Spring Veggies

Servings: 4
Cooking Time: 8 Minutes
Ingredients:
- ½ pound asparagus ends trimmed, cut into 2-inch pieces
- 1 cup sugar snap peas
- 1 pound sea scallops
- 1 tablespoon lemon juice
- 2 teaspoons olive oil
- ½ teaspoon dried thyme
- Pinch salt
- Freshly ground black pepper

Directions:
1. Preparing the Ingredients. Place the asparagus and sugar snap peas in the Oven rack/basket. Place the Rack on the middle-shelf of the air fryer oven.
2. Air Frying. Cook for 2 to 3 minutes or until the vegetables are just starting to get tender.
3. Meanwhile, check the scallops for a small muscle attached to the side, and pull it off and discard.
4. In a medium bowl, toss the scallops with the lemon juice, olive oil, thyme, salt, and pepper. Place into the Oven rack/basket on top of the vegetables. Place the Rack on the middle-shelf of the air fryer oven.
5. Air Frying. Steam for 5 to 7 minutes. Until the scallops are just firm, and the vegetables are tender. Serve immediately.
- **Nutrition Info:** CALORIES: 162; CARBS:10G; FAT: 4G; PROTEIN:22G; FIBER:3G

300.Crispy Crab And Fish Cakes

Servings:4
Cooking Time: 12 Minutes
Ingredients:
- 8 ounces (227 g) imitation crab meat
- 4 ounces (113 g) leftover cooked fish (such as cod, pollock, or haddock)
- 2 tablespoons minced celery
- 2 tablespoons minced green onion
- 2 tablespoons light mayonnaise
- 1 tablespoon plus 2 teaspoons Worcestershire sauce
- ¾ cup crushed saltine cracker crumbs
- 2 teaspoons dried parsley flakes
- 1 teaspoon prepared yellow mustard
- ½ teaspoon garlic powder
- ½ teaspoon dried dill weed, crushed
- ½ teaspoon Old Bay seasoning
- ½ cup panko bread crumbs
- Cooking spray

Directions:

1. Pulse the crab meat and fish in a food processor until finely chopped.
2. Transfer the meat mixture to a large bowl, along with the celery, green onion, mayo, Worcestershire sauce, cracker crumbs, parsley flakes, mustard, garlic powder, dill weed, and Old Bay seasoning. Stir to mix well.
3. Scoop out the meat mixture and form into 8 equal-sized patties with your hands.
4. Place the panko bread crumbs on a plate. Roll the patties in the bread crumbs until they are evenly coated on both sides. Put the patties in the baking pan and spritz them with cooking spray.
5. Slide the baking pan into Rack Position 1, select Convection Bake, set temperature to 390ºF (199ºC), and set time to 12 minutes.
6. Flip the patties halfway through the cooking time.
7. When cooking is complete, they should be golden brown and cooked through. Remove the pan from the oven. Divide the patties among four plates and serve.

301.Spicy Baked Shrimp

Servings: 4
Cooking Time: 8 Minutes
Ingredients:
- 2 lbs shrimp, peeled & deveined
- 1/4 tsp cayenne pepper
- 1 tsp garlic powder
- 2 tbsp chili powder
- 2 tbsp olive oil
- 1 tsp kosher salt

Directions:
1. Fit the oven with the rack in position
2. Toss shrimp with remaining ingredients.
3. Transfer shrimp into the baking pan.
4. Set to bake at 400 F for 13 minutes. After 5 minutes place the baking pan in the preheated oven.
5. Serve and enjoy.
- **Nutrition Info:** Calories 344 Fat 11.5 g Carbohydrates 6.1 g Sugar 0.5 g Protein 52.3 g Cholesterol 478 mg

302.Caesar Shrimp Salad

Servings:4
Cooking Time: 15 Minutes
Ingredients:
- ½ baguette, cut into 1-inch cubes (about 2½ cups)
- 4 tablespoons extra-virgin olive oil, divided
- ¼ teaspoon granulated garlic
- ¼ teaspoon kosher salt
- ¾ cup Caesar dressing, divided
- 2 romaine lettuce hearts, cut in half lengthwise and ends trimmed

- 1 pound (454 g) medium shrimp, peeled and deveined
- 2 ounces (57 g) Parmesan cheese, coarsely grated

Directions:
1. Make the croutons: Put the bread cubes in a medium bowl and drizzle 3 tablespoons of olive oil over top. Season with granulated garlic and salt and toss to coat. Transfer to the air fryer basket in a single layer.
2. Put the air fryer basket on the baking pan and slide into Rack Position 2, select Air Fry, set temperature to 400ºF (205ºC), and set time to 4 minutes.
3. Toss the croutons halfway through the cooking time.
4. When done, remove from the oven and set aside.
5. Brush 2 tablespoons of Caesar dressing on the cut side of the lettuce. Set aside.
6. Toss the shrimp with the ¼ cup of Caesar dressing in a large bowl until well coated. Set aside.
7. Coat the baking pan with the remaining 1 tablespoon of olive oil. Arrange the romaine halves on the coated pan, cut side down. Brush the tops with the remaining 2 tablespoons of Caesar dressing.
8. Slide the baking pan into Rack Position 2, select Roast, set temperature to 375ºF (190ºC), and set time to 10 minutes.
9. After 5 minutes, remove from the oven and flip the romaine halves. Spoon the shrimp around the lettuce. Return the pan to the oven and continue cooking.
10. When done, remove from the oven. If they are not quite cooked through, roast for another 1 minute.
11. On each of four plates, put a romaine half. Divide the shrimp among the plates and top with croutons and grated Parmesan cheese. Serve immediately.

303.Rosemary & Garlic Prawns

Servings:2
Cooking Time: 15 Minutes + Chilling Time
Ingredients:
- 8 large prawns
- 2 garlic cloves, minced
- 1 rosemary sprig, chopped
- 1 tbsp butter, melted
- Salt and black pepper to taste

Directions:
1. Combine garlic, butter, rosemary, salt, and pepper in a bowl. Add in the prawns and mix to coat. Cover the bowl and refrigerate for 1 hour. Preheat on AirFry function to 350 F. Remove the prawns from the fridge and transfer to the frying basket. Cook for 6-8 minutes.

304.Maryland Crab Cakes

Servings: 6
Cooking Time: 10 Minutes
Ingredients:
- Nonstick cooking spray
- 2 eggs
- 1 cup Panko bread crumbs
- 1 stalk celery, chopped
- 3 tbsp. mayonnaise
- 1 tsp Worcestershire sauce
- ¼ cup mozzarella cheese, grated
- 1 tsp Italian seasoning
- 1 tbsp. fresh parsley, chopped
- 1 tsp pepper
- ¾ lb. lump crabmeat, drained

Directions:
1. Place baking pan in position 2 of the oven. Lightly spray the fryer basket with cooking spray.
2. In a large bowl, combine all ingredients except crab meat, mix well.
3. Fold in crab carefully so it retains some chunks. Form mixture into 12 patties.
4. Place patties in a single layer in the fryer basket. Place the basket on the baking pan.
5. Set oven to air fryer on 350°F for 10 minutes. Cook until golden brown, turning over halfway through cooking time. Serve immediately.
- **Nutrition Info:** Calories 172, Total Fat 8g, Saturated Fat 2g, Total Carbs 14g, Net Carbs 13g, Protein 16g, Sugar 1g, Fiber 1g, Sodium 527mg, Potassium 290mg, Phosphorus 201mg

305.Roasted Nicoise Salad

Servings:4
Cooking Time: 15 Minutes
Ingredients:
- 10 ounces (283 g) small red potatoes, quartered
- 8 tablespoons extra-virgin olive oil, divided
- 1 teaspoon kosher salt, divided
- ½ pound (227 g) green beans, trimmed
- 1 pint cherry tomatoes
- 1 teaspoon Dijon mustard
- 3 tablespoons red wine vinegar
- Freshly ground black pepper, to taste
- 1 (9-ounce / 255-g) bag spring greens, washed and dried if needed
- 2 (5-ounce / 142-g) cans oil-packed tuna, drained
- 2 hard-cooked eggs, peeled and quartered
- $^1/_3$ cup kalamata olives, pitted

Directions:
1. In a large bowl, drizzle the potatoes with 1 tablespoon of olive oil and season with ¼

teaspoon of kosher salt. Transfer to the baking pan.
2. Slide the baking pan into Rack Position 2, select Roast, set temperature to 375ºF (190ºC), and set time to 15 minutes.
3. Meanwhile, in a mixing bowl, toss the green beans and cherry tomatoes with 1 tablespoon of olive oil and ¼ teaspoon of kosher salt until evenly coated.
4. After 10 minutes, remove the pan and fold in the green beans and cherry tomatoes. Return the pan to the oven and continue cooking.
5. Meanwhile, make the vinaigrette by whisking together the remaining 6 tablespoons of olive oil, mustard, vinegar, the remaining ½ teaspoon of kosher salt, and black pepper in a small bowl. Set aside.
6. When done, remove from the oven. Allow the vegetables to cool for 5 minutes.
7. Spread out the spring greens on a plate and spoon the tuna into the center of the greens. Arrange the potatoes, green beans, cheery tomatoes, and eggs around the tuna. Serve drizzled with the vinaigrette and scattered with the olives.

306.Spiced Red Snapper

Servings:4
Cooking Time: 10 Minutes
Ingredients:
- 1 teaspoon olive oil
- 1½ teaspoons black pepper
- ¼ teaspoon garlic powder
- ¼ teaspoon thyme
- ⅛ teaspoon cayenne pepper
- 4 (4-ounce / 113-g) red snapper fillets, skin on
- 4 thin slices lemon
- Nonstick cooking spray

Directions:
1. Spritz the baking pan with nonstick cooking spray.
2. In a small bowl, stir together the olive oil, black pepper, garlic powder, thyme, and cayenne pepper. Rub the mixture all over the fillets until completely coated.
3. Lay the fillets, skin-side down, in the baking pan and top each fillet with a slice of lemon.
4. Slide the baking pan into Rack Position 1, select Convection Bake, set temperature to 390ºF (199ºC), and set time to 10 minutes.
5. Flip the fillets halfway through the cooking time.
6. When cooking is complete, the fish should be cooked through. Let the fish cool for 5 minutes and serve.

307.Basil Tomato Salmon

Servings: 2

Cooking Time: 20 Minutes
Ingredients:
- 2 salmon fillets
- 1 tomato, sliced
- 1 tbsp dried basil
- 2 tbsp parmesan cheese, grated
- 1 tbsp olive oil

Directions:
1. Fit the oven with the rack in position
2. Place salmon fillets in a baking dish.
3. Sprinkle basil on top of salmon fillets.
4. Arrange tomato slices on top of salmon fillets. Drizzle with oil and top with cheese.
5. Set to bake at 375 F for 25 minutes. After 5 minutes place the baking dish in the preheated oven.
6. Serve and enjoy.
- **Nutrition Info:** Calories 324 Fat 19.6 g Carbohydrates 1.5 g Sugar 0.8 g Protein 37.1 g Cholesterol 83 mg

308.Parmesan-crusted Salmon Patties

Servings:4
Cooking Time: 13 Minutes
Ingredients:
- 1 pound (454 g) salmon, chopped into ½-inch pieces
- 2 tablespoons coconut flour
- 2 tablespoons grated Parmesan cheese
- 1½ tablespoons milk
- ½ white onion, peeled and finely chopped
- ½ teaspoon butter, at room temperature
- ½ teaspoon chipotle powder
- ½ teaspoon dried parsley flakes
- $^1/_3$ teaspoon ground black pepper
- $^1/_3$ teaspoon smoked cayenne pepper
- 1 teaspoon fine sea salt

Directions:
1. Put all the ingredients for the salmon patties in a bowl and stir to combine well.
2. Scoop out 2 tablespoons of the salmon mixture and shape into a patty with your palm, about ½ inch thick. Repeat until all the mixture is used. Transfer to the refrigerator for about 2 hours until firm.
3. When ready, arrange the salmon patties in the baking pan.
4. Slide the baking pan into Rack Position 1, select Convection Bake, set temperature to 395ºF (202ºC), and set time to 13 minutes.
5. Flip the patties halfway through the cooking time.
6. When cooking is complete, the patties should be golden brown. Remove from the oven and cool for 5 minutes before serving.

309.Parsley Catfish Fillets

Servings:4
Cooking Time: 25 Minutes

Ingredients:
- 4 catfish fillets, rinsed and dried
- ¼ cup seasoned fish fry
- 1 tbsp olive oil
- 1 tbsp fresh parsley, chopped

Directions:
1. Add seasoned fish fry and fillets in a large Ziploc bag; massage well to coat. Place the fillets in the basket and cook for 14-16 minutes at 360 F on AirFry function. Top with parsley.

310.Glazed Tuna And Fruit Kebabs

Servings:4
Cooking Time: 10 Minutes
Ingredients:
- Kebabs:
- 1 pound (454 g) tuna steaks, cut into 1-inch cubes
- ½ cup canned pineapple chunks, drained, juice reserved
- ½ cup large red grapes
- Marinade:
- 1 tablespoon honey
- 1 teaspoon olive oil
- 2 teaspoons grated fresh ginger
- Pinch cayenne pepper
- Special Equipment:
- 4 metal skewers

Directions:
1. Make the kebabs: Thread, alternating tuna cubes, pineapple chunks, and red grapes, onto the metal skewers.
2. Make the marinade: Whisk together the honey, olive oil, ginger, and cayenne pepper in a small bowl. Brush generously the marinade over the kebabs and allow to sit for 10 minutes.
3. When ready, transfer the kebabs to the air fryer basket.
4. Put the air fryer basket on the baking pan and slide into Rack Position 2, select Air Fry, set temperature to 370ºF (188ºC), and set time to 10 minutes.
5. After 5 minutes, remove from the oven and flip the kebabs and brush with the remaining marinade. Return the pan to the oven and continue cooking for an additional 5 minutes.
6. When cooking is complete, the kebabs should reach an internal temperature of 145ºF (63ºC) on a meat thermometer. Remove from the oven and discard any remaining marinade. Serve hot.

311.Fried Calamari

Servings: 6-8
Cooking Time: 7 Minutes
Ingredients:

- ½ tsp. salt
- ½ tsp. Old Bay seasoning
- 1/3 C. plain cornmeal
- ½ C. semolina flour
- ½ C. almond flour
- 5-6 C. olive oil
- 1 ½ pounds baby squid

Directions:
1. Preparing the Ingredients. Rinse squid in cold water and slice tentacles, keeping just ¼-inch of the hood in one piece.
2. Combine 1-2 pinches of pepper, salt, Old Bay seasoning, cornmeal, and both flours together. Dredge squid pieces into flour mixture and place into the air fryer oven.
3. Air Frying. Spray liberally with olive oil. Cook 15 minutes at 345 degrees till coating turns a golden brown.
- **Nutrition Info:** CALORIES: 211; CARBS:55; FAT: 6G; PROTEIN:21G; SUGAR:1G

312.Fired Shrimp With Mayonnaise Sauce

Servings:4
Cooking Time: 7 Minutes
Ingredients:
- Shrimp
- 12 jumbo shrimp
- ½ teaspoon garlic salt
- ¼ teaspoon freshly cracked mixed peppercorns
- Sauce:
- 4 tablespoons mayonnaise
- 1 teaspoon grated lemon rind
- 1 teaspoon Dijon mustard
- 1 teaspoon chipotle powder
- ½ teaspoon cumin powder

Directions:
1. In a medium bowl, season the shrimp with garlic salt and cracked mixed peppercorns.
2. Place the shrimp in the air fryer basket.
3. Put the air fryer basket on the baking pan and slide into Rack Position 2, select Air Fry, set temperature to 395ºF (202ºC), and set time to 7 minutes.
4. After 5 minutes, remove from the oven and flip the shrimp. Return to the oven and continue cooking for 2 minutes more, or until they are pink and no longer opaque.
5. Meanwhile, stir together all the ingredients for the sauce in a small bowl until well mixed.
6. When cooking is complete, remove the shrimp from the oven and serve alongside the sauce.

313.Baked Halibut Steaks With Parsley

Servings: 4
Cooking Time: 10 Minutes
Ingredients:

- 1 pound (454 g) halibut steaks
- ¼ cup vegetable oil
- 2½ tablespoons Worcester sauce
- 2 tablespoons honey
- 2 tablespoons vermouth
- 1 tablespoon freshly squeezed lemon juice
- 1 tablespoon fresh parsley leaves, coarsely chopped
- Salt and pepper, to taste
- 1 teaspoon dried basil

Directions:
1. Put all the ingredients in a large mixing dish and gently stir until the fish is coated evenly. Transfer the fish to the baking pan.
2. Slide the baking pan into Rack Position 1, select Convection Bake, set temperature to 375ºF (190ºC), and set time to 10 minutes.
3. Flip the fish halfway through cooking time.
4. When cooking is complete, the fish should reach an internal temperature of at least 145ºF (63ºC) on a meat thermometer. Remove from the oven and let the fish cool for 5 minutes before serving.

314.Mediterranean Sole

Servings: 6
Cooking Time: 20 Minutes
Ingredients:
- Nonstick cooking spray
- 2 tbsp. olive oil
- 8 scallions, sliced thin
- 2 cloves garlic, diced fine
- 4 tomatoes, chopped
- ½ cup dry white wine
- 2 tbsp. fresh parsley, chopped fine
- 1 tsp oregano
- 1 tsp pepper
- 2 lbs. sole, cut in 6 pieces
- 4 oz. feta cheese, crumbled

Directions:
1. Place the rack in position 1 of the oven. Spray an 8x11-inch baking dish with cooking spray.
2. Heat the oil in a medium skillet over medium heat. Add scallions and garlic and cook until tender, stirring frequently.
3. Add the tomatoes, wine, parsley, oregano, and pepper. Stir to mix. Simmer for 5 minutes, or until sauce thickens. Remove from heat.
4. Pour half the sauce on the bottom of the prepared dish. Lay fish on top then pour remaining sauce over the top. Sprinkle with feta.
5. Set the oven to bake on 400°F for 25 minutes. After 5 minutes, place the baking dish on the rack and cook 15-18 minutes or until fish flakes easily with a fork. Serve immediately.

- **Nutrition Info:** Calories 220, Total Fat 12g, Saturated Fat 4g, Total Carbs 6g, Net Carbs 4g, Protein 22g, Sugar 4g, Fiber 2g, Sodium 631mg, Potassium 540mg, Phosphorus 478mg

315.Breaded Scallops

Servings:4
Cooking Time: 7 Minutes
Ingredients:
- 1 egg
- 3 tablespoons flour
- 1 cup bread crumbs
- 1 pound (454 g) fresh scallops
- 2 tablespoons olive oil
- Salt and black pepper, to taste

Directions:
1. In a bowl, lightly beat the egg. Place the flour and bread crumbs into separate shallow dishes.
2. Dredge the scallops in the flour and shake off any excess. Dip the flour-coated scallops in the beaten egg and roll in the bread crumbs.
3. Brush the scallops generously with olive oil and season with salt and pepper, to taste. Transfer the scallops to the air fryer basket.
4. Put the air fryer basket on the baking pan and slide into Rack Position 2, select Air Fry, set temperature to 360ºF (182ºC), and set time to 7 minutes.
5. Flip the scallops halfway through the cooking time.
6. When cooking is complete, the scallops should reach an internal temperature of just 145ºF (63ºC) on a meat thermometer. Remove from the oven. Let the scallops cool for 5 minutes and serve.

316.Cajun Salmon With Lemon

Servings:1
Cooking Time: 10 Minutes
Ingredients:
- 1 salmon fillet
- ¼ tsp brown sugar
- Juice of ½ lemon
- 1 tbsp cajun seasoning
- 2 lemon wedges
- 1 tbsp fresh parsley, chopped

Directions:
1. Preheat on Bake function to 350 F. Combine sugar and lemon and coat in the salmon. Sprinkle with the Cajun seasoning as well. Place a parchment paper on a baking tray and press Start. Cook for 14-16 minutes. Serve with lemon wedges and chopped parsley.

317.Easy Blackened Shrimp

Servings: 6
Cooking Time: 10 Minutes
Ingredients:
- 1 lb shrimp, deveined
- 1 tbsp olive oil
- 1/4 tsp pepper
- 2 tsp blackened seasoning
- 1/4 tsp salt

Directions:
1. Fit the oven with the rack in position
2. Toss shrimp with oil, pepper, blackened seasoning, and salt.
3. Transfer shrimp into the baking pan.
4. Set to bake at 400 F for 15 minutes. After 5 minutes place the baking pan in the preheated oven.
5. Serve and enjoy.
- **Nutrition Info:** Calories 167 Fat 4.3 g Carbohydrates 10.5 g Sugar 0 g Protein 20.6 g Cholesterol 159 mg

318.Sesame Seeds Coated Fish

Servings:5
Cooking Time: 8 Minutes
Ingredients:
- 3 tablespoons plain flour
- 2 eggs
- ½ cup sesame seeds, toasted
- ½ cup breadcrumbs
- 1/8 teaspoon dried rosemary, crushed
- Pinch of salt
- Pinch of black pepper
- 3 tablespoons olive oil
- 5 frozen fish fillets (white fish of your choice)

Directions:
1. Preparing the Ingredients. In a shallow dish, place flour. In a second shallow dish, beat the eggs. In a third shallow dish, add remaining ingredients except fish fillets and mix till a crumbly mixture forms.
2. Coat the fillets with flour and shake off the excess flour.
3. Next, dip the fillets in the egg.
4. Then coat the fillets with sesame seeds mixture generously.
5. Preheat the air fryer oven to 390 degrees F.
6. Air Frying. Line an Air fryer rack/basket with a piece of foil. Arrange the fillets into prepared basket.
7. Cook for about 14 minutes, flipping once after 10 minutes.

319.Blackened Tuna Steaks

Servings:x
Cooking Time:x
Ingredients:
- 2 Tbsp canola oil
- 4 (8-oz) tuna steaks, preferably sushi-grade
- Blackening Spice:
- ½ cup freshly ground black pepper
- 2 Tbsp kosher salt
- 1 Tbsp cardamom
- 1 Tbsp ground cinnamon
- 1 Tbsp nutmeg
- 1 Tbsp ground cloves
- 1 tsp coriander
- 1 tsp cumin
- 1 tsp cayenne pepper
- ½ tsp celery salt

Directions:
1. First prepare the blackening spice by combining all the spices.
2. Preheat oven.
3. Place oil inside the pot and wait until smoking.
4. Sprinkle blackening mixture on top of both sides of tuna steaks (about
5. -2 Tbsp of blackening spice, depending on how spicy you want your steaks).
6. Add tuna into oven and cook about 3 minutes each side. The tuna should be browned on the outside and rare on the inside.

320.Sweet And Savory Breaded Shrimp

Servings: 2
Cooking Time: 20 Minutes
Ingredients:
- ½ pound of fresh shrimp, peeled from their shells and rinsed
- 2 raw eggs
- ½ cup of breadcrumbs (we like Panko, but any brand or home recipe will do)
- ½ white onion, peeled and rinsed and finely chopped
- 1 teaspoon of ginger-garlic paste
- ½ teaspoon of turmeric powder
- ½ teaspoon of red chili powder
- ½ teaspoon of cumin powder
- ½ teaspoon of black pepper powder
- ½ teaspoon of dry mango powder
- Pinch of salt

Directions:
1. Preparing the Ingredients. Cover the basket of the air fryer oven with a lining of tin foil, leaving the edges uncovered to allow air to circulate through the basket.
2. Preheat the air fryer oven to 350 degrees.
3. In a large mixing bowl, beat the eggs until fluffy and until the yolks and whites are fully combined.
4. Dunk all the shrimp in the egg mixture, fully submerging.
5. In a separate mixing bowl, combine the bread crumbs with all the dry ingredients until evenly blended.

6. One by one, coat the egg-covered shrimp in the mixed dry ingredients so that fully covered, and place on the foil-lined air-fryer basket.
7. Air Frying. Set the air-fryer timer to 20 minutes.
8. Halfway through the cooking time, shake the handle of the air-fryer so that the breaded shrimp jostles inside and fry-coverage is even.
9. After 20 minutes, when the fryer shuts off, the shrimp will be perfectly cooked and their breaded crust golden-brown and delicious! Using tongs, remove from the air fryer oven and set on a serving dish to cool.

321.Seafood Pizza

Servings:x
Cooking Time:x
Ingredients:
- One pizza base
- Grated pizza cheese (mozzarella cheese preferably) for topping
- Some pizza topping sauce
- Use cooking oil for brushing and topping purposes
- ingredients for topping:
- 2 onions chopped
- 2 cups mixed seafood
- 2 capsicums chopped
- 2 tomatoes that have been deseeded and chopped
- 1 tbsp. (optional) mushrooms/corns
- 2 tsp. pizza seasoning
- Some cottage cheese that has been cut into small cubes (optional)

Directions:
1. Put the pizza base in a pre-heated oven for around 5 minutes. (Pre heated to 340 Fahrenheit). Take out the base. Pour some pizza sauce on top of the base at the center. Using a spoon spread the sauce over the base making sure that you leave some gap around the circumference. Grate some mozzarella cheese and sprinkle it over the sauce layer. Take all the vegetables and the seafood and mix them in a bowl. Add some oil and seasoning.
2. Also add some salt and pepper according to taste. Mix them properly. Put this topping over the layer of cheese on the pizza. Now sprinkle some more grated cheese and pizza seasoning on top of this layer. Pre heat the oven at 250 Fahrenheit for around 5 minutes.
3. Open the fry basket and place the pizza inside. Close the basket and keep the fryer at 170 degrees for another 10 minutes. If you feel that it is undercooked you may put it at the same temperature for another 2 minutes or so.

322.Moist & Juicy Baked Cod

Servings: 2
Cooking Time: 10 Minutes
Ingredients:
- 1 lb cod fillets
- 1 1/2 tbsp olive oil
- 3 dashes cayenne pepper
- 1 tbsp fresh lemon juice
- 1/4 tsp salt

Directions:
1. Fit the oven with the rack in position
2. Place fish fillets in a baking pan.
3. Drizzle with oil and lemon juice and sprinkle with cayenne pepper and salt.
4. Set to bake at 400 F for 15 minutes. After 5 minutes place the baking pan in the preheated oven.
5. Serve and enjoy.
- **Nutrition Info:** Calories 275 Fat 12.7 g Carbohydrates 0.4 g Sugar 0.2 g Protein 40.6 g Cholesterol 111 mg

323.Fried Cod Nuggets

Servings: 4
Cooking Time: 25 Minutes
Ingredients:
- 1 ¼ lb cod fillets, cut into 4 to 6 chunks each
- ½ cup flour
- 1 egg
- 1 cup cornflakes
- 1 tbsp olive oil
- Salt and black pepper to taste

Directions:
1. Place the olive oil and cornflakes in a food processor and process until crumbed. Season the fish chunks with salt and pepper. In a bowl, beat the egg along with 1 tbsp of water. Dredge the chunks in flour first, then dip in the egg, and finally coat with cornflakes. Arrange the fish pieces on a lined sheet and cook in your on Air Fry at 350 F for 15 minutes until crispy.

324.Delicious Fried Seafood

Servings: 4
Cooking Time: 15 Minutes
Ingredients:
- 1 lb fresh scallops, mussels, fish fillets, prawns, shrimp
- 2 eggs, lightly beaten
- Salt and black pepper to taste
- 1 cup breadcrumbs mixed with zest of 1 lemon

Directions:
1. Dip each piece of the seafood into the eggs and season with salt and pepper. Coat in the crumbs and spray with oil. Arrange into the frying basket and fit in the baking tray; cook for 10 minutes at 400 F on Air Fry function, turning once halfway through. Serve.

325.Flavorful Herb Salmon

Servings: 4
Cooking Time: 15 Minutes
Ingredients:
- 1 lb salmon fillets
- 1/2 tbsp dried rosemary
- 1 tbsp olive oil
- 1/4 tsp dried basil
- 1 tbsp dried chives
- 1/4 tsp dried thyme
- Pepper
- Salt

Directions:
1. Fit the oven with the rack in position 2.
2. Place salmon skin side down in air fryer basket then place an air fryer basket in baking pan.
3. Mix olive oil, thyme, basil, chives, and rosemary in a small bowl.
4. Brush salmon with oil mixture.
5. Place a baking pan on the oven rack. Set to air fry at 400 F for 15 minutes.
6. Serve and enjoy.
- **Nutrition Info:** Calories 182 Fat 10.6 g Carbohydrates 0.4 g Sugar 0 g Protein 22.1 g Cholesterol 50 mg

326.Panko Crab Sticks With Mayo Sauce

Servings:4
Cooking Time: 12 Minutes
Ingredients:
- Crab Sticks:
- 2 eggs
- 1 cup flour
- $^1/_3$ cup panko bread crumbs
- 1 tablespoon old bay seasoning
- 1 pound (454 g) crab sticks
- Cooking spray
- Mayo Sauce:
- ½ cup mayonnaise
- 1 lime, juiced
- 2 garlic cloves, minced

Directions:
1. In a bowl, beat the eggs. In a shallow bowl, place the flour. In another shallow bowl, thoroughly combine the panko bread crumbs and old bay seasoning.
2. Dredge the crab sticks in the flour, shaking off any excess, then in the beaten eggs, finally press them in the bread crumb mixture to coat well.
3. Arrange the crab sticks in the air fryer basket and spray with cooking spray.
4. Put the air fryer basket on the baking pan and slide into Rack Position 2, select Air Fry, set temperature to 390ºF (199ºC), and set time to 12 minutes.
5. Flip the crab sticks halfway through the cooking time.
6. Meanwhile, make the sauce by whisking together the mayo, lime juice, and garlic in a small bowl.

7. When cooking is complete, remove from the oven. Serve the crab sticks with the mayo sauce on the side.

327.Homemade Fish Sticks

Servings: 8 Fish Sticks
Cooking Time: 8 Minutes
Ingredients:
- 8 ounces (227 g) fish fillets (pollock or cod), cut into ½×3-inch strips
- Salt, to taste (optional)
- ½ cup plain bread crumbs
- Cooking spray

Directions:
1. Season the fish strips with salt to taste, if desired.
2. Place the bread crumbs on a plate. Roll the fish strips in the bread crumbs to coat. Spritz the fish strips with cooking spray.
3. Arrange the fish strips in the air fryer basket in a single layer.
4. Put the air fryer basket on the baking pan and slide into Rack Position 2, select Air Fry, set temperature to 390ºF (199ºC), and set time to 8 minutes.
5. When cooking is complete, they should be golden brown. Remove from the oven and cool for 5 minutes before serving.

328.Fish Club Classic Sandwich

Servings:x
Cooking Time:x
Ingredients:
- 2 slices of white bread
- 1 tbsp. softened butter
- 1 tin tuna
- 1 small capsicum
- For Barbeque Sauce:
- ¼ tbsp. Worcestershire sauce
- ½ tsp. olive oil
- ½ flake garlic crushed
- ¼ cup chopped onion
- ¼ tsp. mustard powder
- ½ tbsp. sugar
- ¼ tbsp. red chili sauce
- 1 tbsp. tomato ketchup
- ½ cup water.
- A pinch of salt and black pepper to taste

Directions:
1. Take the slices of bread and remove the edges. Now cut the slices horizontally. Cook the ingredients for the sauce and wait till it thickens. Now, add the fish to the sauce and stir till it obtains the flavors. Roast the capsicum and peel the skin off. Cut the capsicum into slices.
2. Mix the ingredients together and apply it to the bread slices. Pre-heat the oven for 5 minutes at 300 Fahrenheit.
3. Open the basket of the Fryer and place the prepared Classic Sandwiches in it such that no two Classic Sandwiches are touching

each other. Now keep the fryer at 250 degrees for around 15 minutes. Turn the Classic Sandwiches in between the cooking process to cook both slices. Serve the Classic Sandwiches with tomato ketchup or mint sauce.

329.Tasty Parmesan Shrimp

Servings: 4
Cooking Time: 10 Minutes
Ingredients:
- 1 lb shrimp, peeled and deveined
- 1/4 cup parmesan cheese, grated
- 4 garlic cloves, minced
- 1 tbsp olive oil
- 1/4 tsp oregano
- 1/2 tsp pepper
- 1/2 tsp onion powder
- 1/2 tsp basil

Directions:
1. Fit the oven with the rack in position 2.
2. Add all ingredients into the large bowl and toss well.
3. Add shrimp to the air fryer basket then place an air fryer basket in the baking pan.
4. Place a baking pan on the oven rack. Set to air fry at 350 F for 10 minutes.
5. Serve and enjoy.
- **Nutrition Info:** Calories 189 Fat 6.7 g Carbohydrates 3.4 g Sugar 0.1 g Protein 27.9 g Cholesterol 243 mg

330.Dijon Salmon Fillets

Servings: 4
Cooking Time: 15 Minutes
Ingredients:
- 1 lb salmon fillets
- 2 tbsp Dijon mustard
- 1/4 cup brown sugar
- Pepper
- Salt

Directions:
1. Fit the oven with the rack in position 2.
2. Season salmon fillets with pepper and salt.
3. In a small bowl, mix Dijon mustard and brown sugar.
4. Brush salmon fillets with Dijon mustard mixture.
5. Place salmon fillets in the air fryer basket then place an air fryer basket in the baking pan.
6. Place a baking pan on the oven rack. Set to air fry at 350 F for 15 minutes.
7. Serve and enjoy.
- **Nutrition Info:** Calories 190 Fat 7.3 g Carbohydrates 9.3 g Sugar 8.9 g Protein 22.4 g Cholesterol 50 mg

331.Crispy Cheesy Fish Fingers

Servings: 4
Cooking Time: 20 Minutes
Ingredients:
- Large codfish filet, approximately 6-8 ounces, fresh or frozen and thawed, cut into 1 ½-inch strips
- 2 raw eggs
- ½ cup of breadcrumbs (we like Panko, but any brand or home recipe will do)
- 2 tablespoons of shredded or powdered parmesan cheese
- 1 tablespoons of shredded cheddar cheese
- Pinch of salt and pepper

Directions:
1. Preparing the Ingredients. Cover the basket of the air fryer oven with a lining of tin foil, leaving the edges uncovered to allow air to circulate through the basket.
2. Preheat the air fryer oven to 350 degrees.
3. In a large mixing bowl, beat the eggs until fluffy and until the yolks and whites are fully combined.
4. Dunk all the fish strips in the beaten eggs, fully submerging.
5. In a separate mixing bowl, combine the bread crumbs with the parmesan, cheddar, and salt and pepper, until evenly mixed.
6. One by one, coat the egg-covered fish strips in the mixed dry ingredients so that they're fully covered, and place on the foil-lined Oven rack/basket. Place the Rack on the middle-shelf of the air fryer oven.
7. Air Frying. Set the air-fryer timer to 20 minutes.
8. Halfway through the cooking time, shake the handle of the air-fryer so that the breaded fish jostles inside and fry-coverage is even.
9. After 20 minutes, when the fryer shuts off, the fish strips will be perfectly cooked and their breaded crust golden-brown and delicious! Using tongs, remove from the air fryer oven and set on a serving dish to cool.

332.Delicious Crab Cakes

Servings: 5
Cooking Time: 10 Minutes
Ingredients:
- 18 oz can crab meat, drained
- 2 1/2 tbsp mayonnaise
- 2 eggs, lightly beaten
- 1/4 cup breadcrumbs
- 1 1/2 tsp dried parsley
- 1 tbsp dried celery
- 1 tsp Old bay seasoning
- 1 1/2 tbsp Dijon mustard
- Pepper
- Salt

Directions:
1. Fit the oven with the rack in position 2.
2. Add all ingredients into the mixing bowl and mix until well combined.
3. Make patties from mixture and place in the air fryer basket then place an air fryer basket in the baking pan.

4. Place a baking pan on the oven rack. Set to air fry at 320 F for 10 minutes.
5. Serve and enjoy.
- **Nutrition Info:** Calories 138 Fat 4.7 g Carbohydrates 7.8 g Sugar 2.7 g Protein 16.8 g Cholesterol 127 mg

333.Crispy Crab Legs

Servings: 4
Cooking Time: 15 Minutes
Ingredients:
- 3 pounds crab legs
- ½ cup butter, melted

Directions:
1. Preheat on Air Fry function to 380 F. Cover the crab legs with salted water and let them stay for a few minutes. Drain, pat them dry, and place the legs in the basket. Fit in the baking tray and brush with some butter; cook for 10 minutes, flipping once. Drizzle with the remaining butter and serve.

334.Fish Spicy Lemon Kebab

Servings:x
Cooking Time:x
Ingredients:
- 1 lb. boneless fish roughly chopped
- 3 onions chopped
- 5 green chilies-roughly chopped
- 1 ½ tbsp. ginger paste
- 1 ½ tsp garlic paste
- 1 ½ tsp salt
- 3 tsp lemon juice
- 2 tsp garam masala
- 4 tbsp. chopped coriander
- 3 tbsp. cream
- 2 tbsp. coriander powder
- 4 tbsp. fresh mint chopped
- 3 tbsp. chopped capsicum
- 3 eggs
- 2 ½ tbsp. white sesame seeds

Directions:
1. Take all the ingredients mentioned under the first heading and mix them in a bowl. Grind them thoroughly to make a smooth paste. Take the eggs in a different bowl and beat them. Add a pinch of salt and leave them aside. Take a flat plate and in it mix the sesame seeds and breadcrumbs. Mold the fish mixture into small balls and flatten them into round and flat kebabs. Dip these kebabs in the egg and salt mixture and then in the mixture of breadcrumbs and sesame seeds. Leave these kebabs in the fridge for an hour or so to set.
2. Pre heat the oven at 160 degrees Fahrenheit for around 5 minutes. Place the kebabs in the basket and let them cook for another 25 minutes at the same temperature. Turn the kebabs over in between the cooking process to get a

uniform cook. Serve the kebabs with mint sauce.

335.Lemon Pepper White Fish Fillets

Servings: 2
Cooking Time: 12 Minutes
Ingredients:
- 12 oz white fish fillets
- 1/2 tsp lemon pepper seasoning
- Pepper
- Salt

Directions:
1. Fit the oven with the rack in position 2.
2. Spray fish fillets with cooking spray and season with lemon pepper seasoning, pepper, and salt.
3. Place fish fillets in the air fryer basket then place an air fryer basket in the baking pan.
4. Place a baking pan on the oven rack. Set to air fry at 360 F for 12 minutes.
5. Serve and enjoy.
- **Nutrition Info:** Calories 294 Fat 12.8 g Carbohydrates 0.4 g Sugar 0 g Protein 41.7 g Cholesterol 131 mg

336.Spicy Catfish

Servings: 4
Cooking Time: 15 Minutes
Ingredients:
- 1 lb catfish fillets, cut 1/2-inch thick
- 1 tsp crushed red pepper
- 2 tsp onion powder
- 1 tbsp dried oregano, crushed
- 1/2 tsp ground cumin
- 1/2 tsp chili powder
- Pepper
- Salt

Directions:
1. Fit the oven with the rack in position
2. In a small bowl, mix cumin, chili powder, crushed red pepper, onion powder, oregano, pepper, and salt.
3. Rub fish fillets with the spice mixture and place in baking dish.
4. Set to bake at 350 F for 20 minutes. After 5 minutes place the baking dish in the preheated oven.
5. Serve and enjoy.
- **Nutrition Info:** Calories 164 Fat 8.9 g Carbohydrates 2.3 g Sugar 0.6 g Protein 18 g Cholesterol 53 mg

337.Spicy Orange Shrimp

Servings:4
Cooking Time: 12 Minutes
Ingredients:
- $^1/_3$ cup orange juice
- 3 teaspoons minced garlic
- 1 teaspoon Old Bay seasoning
- ¼ to ½ teaspoon cayenne pepper

- 1 pound (454 g) medium shrimp, thawed, deveined, peeled, with tails off, and patted dry
- Cooking spray

Directions:
1. Stir together the orange juice, garlic, Old Bay seasoning, and cayenne pepper in a medium bowl. Add the shrimp to the bowl and toss to coat well.
2. Cover the bowl with plastic wrap and marinate in the refrigerator for 30 minutes.
3. Spritz the air fryer basket with cooking spray. Place the shrimp in the pan and spray with cooking spray.
4. Put the air fryer basket on the baking pan and slide into Rack Position 2, select Air Fry, set temperature to 400ºF (205ºC), and set time to 12 minutes.
5. Flip the shrimp halfway through the cooking time.
6. When cooked, the shrimp should be opaque and crisp. Remove from the oven and serve hot.

338. Breaded Calamari With Lemon

Servings: 4
Cooking Time: 12 Minutes
Ingredients:
- 2 large eggs
- 2 garlic cloves, minced
- ½ cup cornstarch
- 1 cup bread crumbs
- 1 pound (454 g) calamari rings
- Cooking spray
- 1 lemon, sliced

Directions:
1. In a small bowl, whisk the eggs with minced garlic. Place the cornstarch and bread crumbs into separate shallow dishes.
2. Dredge the calamari rings in the cornstarch, then dip in the egg mixture, shaking off any excess, finally roll them in the bread crumbs to coat well. Let the calamari rings sit for 10 minutes in the refrigerator.
3. Spritz the air fryer basket with cooking spray. Transfer the calamari rings to the pan.
4. Put the air fryer basket on the baking pan and slide into Rack Position 2, select Air Fry, set temperature to 390ºF (199ºC), and set time to 12 minutes.
5. Stir the calamari rings once halfway through the cooking time.
6. When cooking is complete, remove from the oven. Serve the calamari rings with the lemon slices sprinkled on top.

339. Parmesan Fish Fillets

Servings: 4
Cooking Time: 17 Minutes
Ingredients:
- $^1/_3$ cup grated Parmesan cheese
- ½ teaspoon fennel seed
- ½ teaspoon tarragon
- $^1/_3$ teaspoon mixed peppercorns
- 2 eggs, beaten
- 4 (4-ounce / 113-g) fish fillets, halved
- 2 tablespoons dry white wine
- 1 teaspoon seasoned salt

Directions:
1. Place the grated Parmesan cheese, fennel seed, tarragon, and mixed peppercorns in a food processor and pulse for about 20 seconds until well combined. Transfer the cheese mixture to a shallow dish.
2. Place the beaten eggs in another shallow dish.
3. Drizzle the dry white wine over the top of fish fillets. Dredge each fillet in the beaten eggs on both sides, shaking off any excess, then roll them in the cheese mixture until fully coated. Season with the salt.
4. Arrange the fillets in the air fryer basket.
5. Put the air fryer basket on the baking pan and slide into Rack Position 2, select Air Fry, set temperature to 345ºF (174ºC), and set time to 17 minutes.
6. Flip the fillets once halfway through the cooking time.
7. When cooking is complete, the fish should be cooked through no longer translucent. Remove from the oven and cool for 5 minutes before serving.

340. Garlic-butter Shrimp With Vegetables

Servings: 4
Cooking Time: 15 Minutes
Ingredients:
- 1 pound (454 g) small red potatoes, halved
- 2 ears corn, shucked and cut into rounds, 1 to 1½ inches thick
- 2 tablespoons Old Bay or similar seasoning
- ½ cup unsalted butter, melted
- 1 (12- to 13-ounce / 340- to 369-g) package kielbasa or other smoked sausages
- 3 garlic cloves, minced
- 1 pound (454 g) medium shrimp, peeled and deveined

Directions:
1. Place the potatoes and corn in a large bowl.
2. Stir together the butter and Old Bay seasoning in a small bowl. Drizzle half the butter mixture over the potatoes and corn, tossing to coat. Spread out the vegetables in the baking pan.
3. Slide the baking pan into Rack Position 2, select Roast, set temperature to 350ºF (180ºC), and set time to 15 minutes.
4. Meanwhile, cut the sausages into 2-inch lengths, then cut each piece in half lengthwise. Put the sausages and shrimp in a medium bowl and set aside.
5. Add the garlic to the bowl of remaining butter mixture and stir well.
6. After 10 minutes, remove the pan and pour the vegetables into the large bowl. Drizzle

with the garlic butter and toss until well coated. Arrange the vegetables, sausages, and shrimp in the pan.
7. Return to the oven and continue cooking. After 5 minutes, check the shrimp for doneness. The shrimp should be pink and opaque. If they are not quite cooked through, roast for an additional 1 minute.
8. When done, remove from the oven and serve on a plate.

341.Garlic Shrimp With Parsley

Servings:4
Cooking Time: 5 Minutes
Ingredients:
- 18 shrimp, shelled and deveined
- 2 garlic cloves, peeled and minced
- 2 tablespoons extra-virgin olive oil
- 2 tablespoons freshly squeezed lemon juice
- ½ cup fresh parsley, coarsely chopped
- 1 teaspoon onion powder
- 1 teaspoon lemon-pepper seasoning
- ½ teaspoon hot paprika
- ½ teaspoon salt
- ¼ teaspoon cumin powder

Directions:
1. Toss all the ingredients in a mixing bowl until the shrimp are well coated.
2. Cover and allow to marinate in the refrigerator for 30 minutes.
3. When ready, transfer the shrimp to the air fryer basket.
4. Put the air fryer basket on the baking pan and slide into Rack Position 2, select Air Fry, set temperature to 400ºF (205ºC), and set time to 5 minutes.
5. When cooking is complete, the shrimp should be pink on the outside and opaque in the center. Remove from the oven and serve warm.

342.Parmesan-crusted Hake With Garlic Sauce

Servings:3

Cooking Time: 10 Minutes
Ingredients:
- Fish:
- 6 tablespoons mayonnaise
- 1 tablespoon fresh lime juice
- 1 teaspoon Dijon mustard
- 1 cup grated Parmesan cheese
- Salt, to taste
- ¼ teaspoon ground black pepper, or more to taste
- 3 hake fillets, patted dry
- Nonstick cooking spray
- Garlic Sauce:
- ¼ cup plain Greek yogurt
- 2 tablespoons olive oil
- 2 cloves garlic, minced
- ½ teaspoon minced tarragon leaves

Directions:
1. Mix the mayo, lime juice, and mustard in a shallow bowl and whisk to combine. In another shallow bowl, stir together the grated Parmesan cheese, salt, and pepper.
2. Dredge each fillet in the mayo mixture, then roll them in the cheese mixture until they are evenly coated on both sides.
3. Spray the air fryer basket with nonstick cooking spray. Place the fillets in the pan.
4. Put the air fryer basket on the baking pan and slide into Rack Position 2, select Air Fry, set temperature to 395ºF (202ºC), and set time to 10 minutes.
5. Flip the fillets halfway through the cooking time.
6. Meanwhile, in a small bowl, whisk all the ingredients for the sauce until well incorporated.
7. When cooking is complete, the fish should flake apart with a fork. Remove the fillets from the oven and serve warm alongside the sauce.

MEATLESS RECIPES

343.Mushroom Pasta

Servings:x
Cooking Time:x
Ingredients:

- 2 cups sliced mushroom
- 2 tbsp. all-purpose flour
- 2 cups of milk
- 1 tsp. dried oregano
- ½ tsp. dried basil
- ½ tsp. dried parsley
- 1 cup pasta
- 1 ½ tbsp. olive oil
- A pinch of salt
- For tossing pasta:
- 1 ½ tbsp. olive oil
- Salt and pepper to taste
- ½ tsp. oregano
- ½ tsp. basil
- 2 tbsp. olive oil
- Salt and pepper to taste

Directions:
1. Boil the pasta and sieve it when done. You will need to toss the pasta in the ingredients mentioned above and set aside.
2. For the sauce, add the ingredients to a pan and bring the ingredients to a boil. Stir the sauce and continue to simmer to make a thicker sauce. Add the pasta to the sauce and transfer this into a glass bowl garnished with cheese.
3. Pre heat the oven at 160 degrees for 5 minutes. Place the bowl in the basket and close it. Let it continue to cook at the same temperature for 10 minutes more. Keep stirring the pasta in between.

344.Maple And Pecan Granola

Servings:4
Cooking Time: 20 Minutes
Ingredients:

- 1½ cups rolled oats
- ¼ cup maple syrup
- ¼ cup pecan pieces
- 1 teaspoon vanilla extract
- ½ teaspoon ground cinnamon

Directions:
1. Line a baking sheet with parchment paper.
2. Mix together the oats, maple syrup, pecan pieces, vanilla, and cinnamon in a large bowl and stir until the oats and pecan pieces are completely coated. Spread the mixture evenly in the baking pan.
3. Slide the baking pan into Rack Position 1, select Convection Bake, set temperature to 300ºF (150ºC), and set time to 20 minutes.
4. Stir once halfway through the cooking time.

5. When done, remove from the oven and cool for 30 minutes before serving. The granola may still be a bit soft right after removing, but it will gradually firm up as it cools.

345.Roasted Vegetables Salad

Servings: 5
Cooking Time: 85 Minutes
Ingredients:

- 3 eggplants
- 1 tbsp of olive oil
- 3 medium zucchini
- 1 tbsp of olive oil
- 4 large tomatoes, cut them in eighths
- 4 cups of one shaped pasta
- 2 peppers of any color
- 1 cup of sliced tomatoes cut into small cubes
- 2 teaspoon of salt substitute
- 8 tbsp of grated parmesan cheese
- ½ cup of Italian dressing
- Leaves of fresh basil

Directions:
1. Preparing the Ingredients. Wash your eggplant and slice it off then discard the green end. Make sure not to peel.
2. Slice your eggplant into1/2 inch of thick rounds. 1/2 inch)
3. Pour 1tbsp of olive oil on the eggplant round.
4. Air Frying. Put the eggplants in the basket of the air fryer oven and then toss it in the air fryer oven. Cook the eggplants for 40 minutes. Set the heat to 360 ° F
5. Meanwhile, wash your zucchini and slice it then discard the green end. But do not peel it.
6. Slice the Zucchini into thick rounds of ½ inch each. Toss your ingredients
7. Add 1 tbsp of olive oil.
8. Air Frying. Cook the zucchini for 25 minutes on a heat of 360° F and when the time is off set it aside.
9. Wash and cut the tomatoes.
10. Air Frying. Arrange your tomatoes in the basket of the air fryer oven. Set the timer to 30 minutes. Set the heat to 350° F
11. When the time is off, cook your pasta according to the pasta guiding directions, empty it into a colander. Run the cold water on it and wash it and drain the pasta and put it aside.
12. Meanwhile, wash and chop your peppers and place it in a bow
13. Wash and thinly slice your cherry tomatoes and add it to the bowl. Add your roasted veggies.

14. Add the pasta, a pinch of salt, the topping dressing, add the basil and the parm and toss everything together. (It is better to mix with your hands). Set the ingredients together in the refrigerator, and let it chill
15. Serve your salad and enjoy it!

346.Lemony Wax Beans

Servings:4
Cooking Time: 12 Minutes
Ingredients:
- 2 pounds (907 g) wax beans
- 2 tablespoons extra-virgin olive oil
- Salt and freshly ground black pepper, to taste
- Juice of ½ lemon, for serving

Directions:
1. Line the air fryer basket with aluminum foil.
2. Toss the wax beans with the olive oil in a large bowl. Lightly season with salt and pepper.
3. Spread out the wax beans in the basket.
4. Put the air fryer basket on the baking pan and slide into Rack Position 2, select Roast, set temperature to 400ºF (205ºC), and set time to 12 minutes.
5. When done, the beans will be caramelized and tender. Remove from the oven to a plate and serve sprinkled with the lemon juice.

347.Stuffed Mushrooms

Servings: 12
Cooking Time: 8 Minutes
Ingredients:
- 2 Rashers Bacon, Diced
- ½ Onion, Diced
- ½ Bell Pepper, Diced
- 1 Small Carrot, Diced
- 24 Medium Size Mushrooms (Separate the caps & stalks)
- 1 cup Shredded Cheddar Plus Extra for the Top
- ½ cup Sour Cream

Directions:
1. Preparing the Ingredients. Chop the mushrooms stalks finely and fry them up with the bacon, onion, pepper and carrot at 350 ° for 8 minutes.
2. When the veggies are fairly tender, stir in the sour cream & the cheese. Keep on the heat until the cheese has melted and everything is mixed nicely.
3. Now grab the mushroom caps and heap a plop of filling on each one.
4. Place in the fryer basket and top with a little extra cheese.

348.Banana Best Homemade Croquette

Servings:x
Cooking Time:x
Ingredients:
- 2 tsp. garam masala
- 4 tbsp. chopped coriander
- 3 tbsp. cream
- 3 tbsp. chopped capsicum
- 3 eggs
- 2 ½ tbsp. white sesame seeds
- 2 cups sliced banana
- 3 onions chopped
- 5 green chilies-roughly chopped
- 1 ½ tbsp. ginger paste
- 1 ½ tsp. garlic paste
- 1 ½ tsp. salt
- 3 tsp. lemon juice

Directions:
1. Grind the ingredients except for the egg and form a smooth paste. Coat the banana in the paste. Now, beat the eggs and add a little salt to it.
2. Dip the coated bananas in the egg mixture and then transfer to the sesame seeds and coat the vegetables well. Place the vegetables on a stick.
3. Pre heat the oven at 160 degrees Fahrenheit for around 5 minutes. Place the sticks in the basket and let them cook for another 25 minutes at the same temperature. Turn the sticks over in between the cooking process to get a uniform cook.

349.Korean Tempeh Steak With Broccoli

Servings: 4
Cooking Time: 15 Minutes + Marinating Time
Ingredients:
- 16 oz tempeh, cut into 1 cm thick pieces
- 1 pound broccoli, cut into florets
- ⅓ cup fermented soy sauce
- 2 tbsp sesame oil
- ⅓ cup sherry
- 1 tsp soy sauce
- 1 tsp white sugar
- 1 tsp cornstarch
- 1 tbsp olive oil
- 1 garlic clove, minced

Directions:
1. In a bowl, mix cornstarch, sherry, fermented soy sauce, sesame oil, soy sauce, sugar, and tempeh pieces. Marinate for 45 minutes.
2. Then, add in garlic, olive oil, and ginger. Place in the basket and fit in the baking tray; cook for 10 minutes at 390 F on Air Fry function, turning once halfway through. Serve.

350.Crispy Eggplant Slices With Parsley

Servings:4
Cooking Time: 12 Minutes
Ingredients:
- 1 cup flour
- 4 eggs
- Salt, to taste
- 2 cups bread crumbs
- 1 teaspoon Italian seasoning
- 2 eggplants, sliced
- 2 garlic cloves, sliced
- 2 tablespoons chopped parsley
- Cooking spray

Directions:
1. Spritz the air fryer basket with cooking spray. Set aside.
2. On a plate, place the flour. In a shallow bowl, whisk the eggs with salt. In another shallow bowl, combine the bread crumbs and Italian seasoning.
3. Dredge the eggplant slices, one at a time, in the flour, then in the whisked eggs, finally in the bread crumb mixture to coat well.
4. Lay the coated eggplant slices in the basket.
5. Put the air fryer basket on the baking pan and slide into Rack Position 2, select Air Fry, set temperature to 390ºF (199ºC), and set time to 12 minutes.
6. Flip the eggplant slices halfway through the cooking time.
7. When cooking is complete, the eggplant slices should be golden brown and crispy. Transfer the eggplant slices to a plate and sprinkle the garlic and parsley on top before serving.

351.Cottage Cheese Pops

Servings:x
Cooking Time:x
Ingredients:
- 1 tsp. dry basil
- ½ cup hung curd
- 1 tsp. lemon juice
- 1 cup cottage cheese cut into 2" cubes
- 1 ½ tsp. garlic paste
- Salt and pepper to taste
- 1 tsp. dry oregano
- 1 tsp. red chili flakes

Directions:
1. Cut the cottage cheese into thick and long rectangular pieces.
2. Add the rest of the ingredients into a separate bowl and mix them well to get a consistent mixture.
3. Dip the cottage cheese pieces in the above mixture and leave them aside for some time.
4. Pre heat the oven at 180° C for around 5 minutes. Place the coated cottage cheese pieces in the fry basket and close it properly.

Let them cook at the same temperature for 20 more minutes. Keep turning them over in the basket so that they are cooked properly. Serve with tomato ketchup.

352.Sesame-thyme Whole Maitake Mushrooms

Servings:2
Cooking Time: 15 Minutes
Ingredients:
- 1 tablespoon soy sauce
- 2 teaspoons toasted sesame oil
- 3 teaspoons vegetable oil, divided
- 1 garlic clove, minced
- 7 ounces (198 g) maitake (hen of the woods) mushrooms
- ½ teaspoon flaky sea salt
- ½ teaspoon sesame seeds
- ½ teaspoon finely chopped fresh thyme leaves

Directions:
1. Whisk together the soy sauce, sesame oil, 1 teaspoon of vegetable oil, and garlic in a small bowl.
2. Arrange the mushrooms in the air fryer basket in a single layer. Drizzle the soy sauce mixture over the mushrooms.
3. Put the air fryer basket on the baking pan and slide into Rack Position 2, select Roast, set temperature to 300ºF (150ºC), and set time to 15 minutes.
4. After 10 minutes, remove from the oven. Flip the mushrooms and sprinkle the sea salt, sesame seeds, and thyme leaves on top. Drizzle the remaining 2 teaspoons of vegetable oil all over. Return to the oven and continue roasting for an additional 5 minutes.
5. When cooking is complete, remove the mushrooms from the oven to a plate and serve hot.

353.Cottage Cheese French Cuisine Galette

Servings:x
Cooking Time:x
Ingredients:
- 1-2 tbsp. fresh coriander leaves
- 2 or 3 green chilies finely chopped
- 1 ½ tbsp. lemon juice
- Salt and pepper to taste
- 2 tbsp. garam masala
- 2 cups grated cottage cheese
- 1 ½ cup coarsely crushed peanuts
- 3 tsp. ginger finely chopped

Directions:
1. Mix the ingredients in a clean bowl.
2. Mold this mixture into round and flat French Cuisine Galettes.

3. Wet the French Cuisine Galettes slightly with water. Coat each French Cuisine Galette with the crushed peanuts.
4. Pre heat the oven at 160 degrees Fahrenheit for 5 minutes. Place the French Cuisine Galettes in the fry basket and let them cook for another 25 minutes at the same temperature. Keep rolling them over to get a uniform cook. Serve either with mint sauce or ketchup.

354.Mushroom French Cuisine Galette

Servings:x
Cooking Time:x
Ingredients:
- 2 or 3 green chilies finely chopped
- 1 ½ tbsp. lemon juice
- Salt and pepper to taste
- 2 tbsp. garam masala
- 2 cups sliced mushrooms
- 1 ½ cup coarsely crushed peanuts
- 3 tsp. ginger finely chopped
- 1-2 tbsp. fresh coriander leaves

Directions:
1. Mix the ingredients in a clean bowl.
2. Mold this mixture into round and flat French Cuisine Galettes.
3. Wet the French Cuisine Galettes slightly with water. Coat each French Cuisine Galette with the crushed peanuts.
4. Pre heat the oven at 160 degrees Fahrenheit for 5 minutes. Place the French Cuisine Galettes in the fry basket and let them cook for another 25 minutes at the same temperature. Keep rolling them over to get a uniform cook. Serve either with mint sauce or ketchup.

355.Crispy Veggies With Halloumi

Servings:2
Cooking Time: 14 Minutes
Ingredients:
- 2 zucchinis, cut into even chunks
- 1 large eggplant, peeled, cut into chunks
- 1 large carrot, cut into chunks
- 6 ounces (170 g) halloumi cheese, cubed
- 2 teaspoons olive oil
- Salt and black pepper, to taste
- 1 teaspoon dried mixed herbs

Directions:
1. Combine the zucchinis, eggplant, carrot, cheese, olive oil, salt, and pepper in a large bowl and toss to coat well.
2. Spread the mixture evenly in the air fryer basket.
3. Put the air fryer basket on the baking pan and slide into Rack Position 2, select Air Fry, set temperature to 340ºF (171ºC), and set time to 14 minutes.

4. Stir the mixture once during cooking.
5. When cooking is complete, they should be crispy and golden. Remove from the oven and serve topped with mixed herbs.

356.Cheesy Ravioli Lunch

Servings:6
Cooking Time: 15 Minutes
Ingredients:
- 1 package cheese ravioli
- 2 cup Italian breadcrumbs
- ¼ cup Parmesan cheese, grated
- 1 cup buttermilk
- 1 tsp olive oil
- ¼ tsp garlic powder

Directions:
1. Preheat on AirFry function to 390 F. In a bowl, combine breadcrumbs, Parmesan cheese, garlic, and olive oil. Dip the ravioli in the buttermilk and coat with the breadcrumb mixture.
2. Line a baking sheet with parchment paper and arrange the ravioli on it. Press Start and cook for 5 minutes. Serve with marinara jar sauce.

357.Balsamic Asparagus

Servings:4
Cooking Time: 10 Minutes
Ingredients:
- 4 tablespoons olive oil, plus more for greasing
- 4 tablespoons balsamic vinegar
- 1½ pounds (680 g) asparagus spears, trimmed
- Salt and freshly ground black pepper, to taste

Directions:
1. Grease the air fryer basket with olive oil.
2. In a shallow bowl, stir together the 4 tablespoons of olive oil and balsamic vinegar to make a marinade.
3. Put the asparagus spears in the bowl so they are thoroughly covered by the marinade and allow to marinate for 5 minutes.
4. Put the asparagus in the greased basket in a single layer and season with salt and pepper.
5. Put the air fryer basket on the baking pan and slide into Rack Position 2, select Air Fry, set temperature to 350ºF (180ºC), and set time to 10 minutes.
6. Flip the asparagus halfway through the cooking time.
7. When done, the asparagus should be tender and lightly browned. Cool for 5 minutes before serving.

358.Feta & Scallion Triangles

Servings:4
Cooking Time: 20 Minutes
Ingredients:
- 4 oz feta cheese, crumbled
- 2 sheets filo pastry
- 1 egg yolk, beaten
- 2 tbsp fresh parsley, finely chopped
- 1 scallion, finely chopped
- 2 tbsp olive oil
- Salt and black pepper to taste

Directions:
1. In a bowl, mix the yolk with the cheese, parsley, and scallion. Season with salt and black pepper. Cut each filo sheet in 3 strips. Put a teaspoon of the feta mixture on the bottom. Roll the strip in a spinning spiral way until the filling of the inside mixture is completely wrapped in a triangle.
2. Preheat on Bake function to 360 F. Brush the surface of filo with olive oil. Place up to 5 triangles in the oven and press Start. Cook for 5 minutes. Lower the temperature to 330 F, cook for 3 more minutes or until golden brown.

359.Winter Vegetarian Frittata

Servings: 4
Cooking Time: 30 Minutes
Ingredients:
- 1 leek, peeled and thinly sliced into rings
- 2 cloves garlic, finely minced
- 3 medium-sized carrots, finely chopped
- 2 tablespoons olive oil
- 6 large-sized eggs
- Sea salt and ground black pepper, to taste
- 1/2 teaspoon dried marjoram, finely minced
- 1/2 cup yellow cheese of choice

Directions:
1. Preparing the Ingredients. Sauté the leek, garlic, and carrot in hot olive oil until they are tender and fragrant; reserve.
2. In the meantime, preheat your air fryer oven to 330 degrees F.
3. In a bowl, whisk the eggs along with the salt, ground black pepper, and marjoram.
4. Then, grease the inside of your baking dish with a nonstick cooking spray. Pour the whisked eggs into the baking dish. Stir in the sautéed carrot mixture. Top with the cheese shreds.
5. Air Frying. Place the baking dish in the air fryer oven cooking basket. Cook about 30 minutes and serve warm

360.Rosemary Butternut Squash Roast

Servings: 2
Cooking Time: 30 Minutes

Ingredients:
- 1 butternut squash
- 1 tbsp dried rosemary
- 2 tbsp maple syrup
- Salt to taste

Directions:
1. Place the squash on a cutting board and peel. Cut in half and remove the seeds and pulp. Slice into wedges and season with salt. Preheat on Air Fry function to 350 F. Spray the wedges with cooking spray and sprinkle with rosemary. Place the wedges in the basket without overlapping and fit in the baking tray. Cook for 20 minutes, flipping once halfway through. Serve with maple syrup and goat cheese.

361.Vegan Beetroot Chips

Servings:2
Cooking Time: 9 Minutes
Ingredients:
- 4 cups golden beetroot slices
- 2 tbsp olive oil
- 1 tbsp yeast flakes
- 1 tsp vegan seasoning
- Salt to taste

Directions:
1. In a bowl, add the oil, beetroot slices, vegan seasoning, and yeast and mix well. Dump the coated chips in the basket. Set the heat to 370 F and press Start. Cook on AirFry function for14-16 minutes, shaking once halfway through. Serve.

362.Potato Wedges

Servings:x
Cooking Time:x
Ingredients:
- 1 tsp. mixed herbs
- ½ tsp. red chili flakes
- A pinch of salt to taste
- 1 tbsp. lemon juice
- 2 medium sized potatoes (Cut into wedges)
- ingredients for the marinade:
- 1 tbsp. olive oil

Directions:
1. Boil the potatoes and blanch them. Mix the ingredients for the marinade and add the potato Oregano Fingers to it making sure that they are coated well.
2. Pre heat the oven for around 5 minutes at 300 Fahrenheit. Take out the basket of the fryer and place the potato Oregano Fingers in them. Close the basket.
3. Now keep the fryer at 200 Fahrenheit for 20 or 25 minutes. In between the process, toss the fries twice or thrice so that they get cooked properly.

363.Easy Cheesy Vegetable Quesadilla

Servings:1
Cooking Time: 10 Minutes
Ingredients:
- 1 teaspoon olive oil
- 2 flour tortillas
- ¼ zucchini, sliced
- ¼ yellow bell pepper, sliced
- ¼ cup shredded gouda cheese
- 1 tablespoon chopped cilantro
- ½ green onion, sliced

Directions:
1. Coat the air fryer basket with 1 teaspoon of olive oil.
2. Arrange a flour tortilla in the basket and scatter the top with zucchini, bell pepper, gouda cheese, cilantro, and green onion. Place the other flour tortilla on top.
3. Put the air fryer basket on the baking pan and slide into Rack Position 2, select Air Fry, set temperature to 390ºF (199ºC), and set time to 10 minutes.
4. When cooking is complete, the tortillas should be lightly browned and the vegetables should be tender. Remove from the oven and cool for 5 minutes before slicing into wedges.

364.Mushrooms Stuffed With Tempeh & Cheddar

Servings:4
Cooking Time: 20 Minutes
Ingredients:
- 14 small button mushrooms
- 1 garlic clove, minced
- Salt and black pepper to taste
- 4 slices tempeh, chopped
- ¼ cup cheddar cheese, grated
- 1 tbsp olive oil
- 1 tbsp fresh parsley, chopped

Directions:
1. Preheat on AirFry function to 390 F. In a bowl, mix the oil, tempeh, cheddar cheese, parsley, salt, pepper, and garlic. Cut the mushroom stalks off and fill them with the tempeh mixture. Place the stuffed mushrooms in the basket and press Start. Cook at 390 F for 8 minutes. Once golden and crispy, plate them and serve with a green salad.

365.Aloo Patties

Servings:x
Cooking Time:x
Ingredients:
- 1 tbsp. fresh coriander leaves
- ¼ tsp. red chili powder
- ¼ tsp. cumin powder

- 1 cup mashed potato
- A pinch of salt to taste
- ¼ tsp. ginger finely chopped
- 1 green chili finely chopped
- 1 tsp. lemon juice

Directions:
1. Mix the ingredients together and ensure that the flavors are right. You will now make round patties with the mixture and roll them out well.
2. Pre heat the oven at 250 Fahrenheit for 5 minutes. Open the basket of the Fryer and arrange the patties in the basket. Close it carefully. Keep the fryer at 150 degrees for around 10 or 12 minutes. In between the cooking process, turn the patties over to get a uniform cook. Serve hot with mint sauce.

366.Parmesan Coated Green Beans

Servings:4
Cooking Time: 20 Minutes
Ingredients:
- 1 cup panko breadcrumbs
- 2 whole eggs, beaten
- ½ cup Parmesan cheese, grated
- ½ cup flour
- 1 tsp cayenne pepper powder
- 1 ½ pounds green beans
- Salt to taste

Directions:
1. Preheat on AirFry function to 380 F. In a bowl, mix breadcrumbs, Parmesan cheese, cayenne pepper powder, salt, and pepper. Flour the green beans and dip them in eggs. Dredge beans in the Parmesan-panko mix. Place in the cooking basket and cook for 15 minutes Serve.

367.Cheese And Mushroom Spicy Lemon Kebab

Servings:x
Cooking Time:x
Ingredients:
- 1-2 tbsp. all-purpose flour for coating purposes
- 1-2 tbsp. mint
- 1 cup molten cheese
- 1 onion that has been finely chopped
- ½ cup milk
- 2 cups sliced mushrooms
- 1-2 green chilies chopped finely
- ¼ tsp. red chili powder
- A pinch of salt to taste
- ½ tsp. dried mango powder
- ¼ tsp. black salt

Directions:
1. Take the mushroom slices and add the grated ginger and the cut green chilies.

Grind this mixture until it becomes a thick paste.

2. Keep adding water as and when required. Now add the onions, mint, the breadcrumbs and all the various masalas required. Mix this well until you get a soft dough. Now take small balls of this mixture (about the size of a lemon) and mold them into the shape of flat and round kebabs. Here is where the milk comes into play.
3. Pour a very small amount of milk onto each kebab to wet it. Now roll the kebab in the dry breadcrumbs. Pre heat the oven for 5 minutes at 300 Fahrenheit. Take out the basket. Arrange the kebabs in the basket leaving gaps between them so that no two kebabs are touching each other. Keep the fryer at 340 Fahrenheit for around half an hour.
4. Half way through the cooking process, turn the kebabs over so that they can be cooked properly. Recommended sides for this dish are mint sauce, tomato ketchup or yoghurt sauce.

368.Portobello Steaks

Servings: 4
Cooking Time: 20 Minutes
Ingredients:
- Nonstick cooking spray
- ¼ cup olive oil
- 2 tbsp. steak seasoning, unsalted
- 1 rosemary stem
- 4 Portobello mushrooms, large caps with stems removed

Directions:
1. Place baking pan in position 2 and spray with cooking spray.
2. In a large bowl, stir together oil, steak seasoning, and rosemary.
3. Add mushrooms and toss to coat all sides thoroughly.
4. Set oven to bake on 400°F for 25 minutes. After 5 minutes, place the mushrooms on the pan and bake 20 minutes, or until mushrooms are tender. Serve immediately.
- **Nutrition Info:** Calories 142, Total Fat 14g, Saturated Fat 2g, Total Carbs 3g, Net Carbs 2g, Protein 1g, Sugar 1g, Fiber 1g, Sodium 309mg, Potassium 118mg, Phosphorus 20mg

369.Vegetable Pie

Servings:x
Cooking Time:x
Ingredients:
- 2 cups roasted vegetables
- 2 tbsp. sugar
- ½ tsp. cinnamon
- 2 tsp. lemon juice

- 1 cup plain flour
- 1 tbsp. unsalted butter
- 4tsp. powdered sugar
- 2 cups cold milk
- ½ cup roasted nuts

Directions:
1. In a large bowl, mix the flour, butter and sugar with your Oregano Fingers. The mixture should resemble breadcrumbs.
2. Squeeze the dough using the cold milk and wrap it and leave it to cool for ten minutes. Now, roll the dough out and cut into two circles.
3. Press the dough into the pie tins and prick on all sides using a fork. Cook the ingredients for the filling on a low flame and pour into the tin. Cover the pie tin with the second round. Preheat the fryer to 300 Fahrenheit for five minutes.
4. You will need to place the tin in the basket and cover it. When the pastry has turned golden brown, you will need to remove the tin and let it cool. Cut into slices and serve with a dollop of cream.

370.Cabbage Fritters(1)

Servings:x
Cooking Time:x
Ingredients:
- 1-2 tbsp. fresh coriander leaves
- 2 or 3 green chilies finely chopped
- 1 ½ tbsp. lemon juice
- Salt and pepper to taste
- 2 tbsp. garam masala
- 2 cups cabbage
- 1 ½ cup coarsely crushed peanuts
- 3 tsp. ginger finely chopped

Directions:
1. Mix the ingredients in a clean bowl.
2. Mold this mixture into round and flat fritters.
3. Wet the fritters slightly with water. Coat each fritter with the crushed peanuts.
4. Pre heat the oven at 160 degrees Fahrenheit for 5 minutes. Place the fritters in the fry basket and let them cook for another 25 minutes at the same temperature. Keep rolling them over to get a uniform cook. Serve either with mint sauce or ketchup.

371.Cornflakes French Toast

Servings:x
Cooking Time:x
Ingredients:
- 1 tsp. sugar for every 2 slices
- Crushed cornflakes
- Bread slices (brown or white)
- 1 egg white for every 2 slices

Directions:
1. Put two slices together and cut them along the diagonal.
2. In a bowl, whisk the egg whites and add some sugar.
3. Dip the bread triangles into this mixture and then coat them with the crushed cornflakes.
4. Pre heat the oven at 180° C for 4 minutes. Place the coated bread triangles in the fry basket and close it. Let them cook at the same temperature for another 20 minutes at least. Halfway through the process, turn the triangles over so that you get a uniform cook. Serve these slices with chocolate sauce.

372. Sweet Baby Carrots

Servings: 4
Cooking Time: 20 Minutes
Ingredients:
- 1 pound baby carrots
- 1 tsp dried dill
- 1 tbsp olive oil
- 1 tbsp honey
- Salt and black pepper to taste

Directions:
1. Preheat your Oven to 300 F on Air Fry function. In a bowl, mix oil, carrots, and honey; gently stir to coat. Season with dill, pepper, and salt. Place the carrots in the cooking basket and fit in the baking tray; cook for 15 minutes, shaking once. Serve.

373. Teriyaki Cauliflower

Servings: 4
Cooking Time: 14 Minutes
Ingredients:
- ½ cup soy sauce
- $^1/_3$ cup water
- 1 tablespoon brown sugar
- 1 teaspoon sesame oil
- 1 teaspoon cornstarch
- 2 cloves garlic, chopped
- ½ teaspoon chili powder
- 1 big cauliflower head, cut into florets

Directions:
1. Make the teriyaki sauce: In a small bowl, whisk together the soy sauce, water, brown sugar, sesame oil, cornstarch, garlic, and chili powder until well combined.
2. Place the cauliflower florets in a large bowl and drizzle the top with the prepared teriyaki sauce and toss to coat well.
3. Put the cauliflower florets in the air fryer basket.
4. Put the air fryer basket on the baking pan and slide into Rack Position 2, select Air Fry,

set temperature to 340ºF (171ºC) and set time to 14 minutes.
5. Stir the cauliflower halfway through.
6. When cooking is complete, the cauliflower should be crisp-tender.
7. Let the cauliflower cool for 5 minutes before serving.

374. Garlicky Vermouth Mushrooms

Servings: 4
Cooking Time: 20 Minutes
Ingredients:
- 2 lb portobello mushrooms, sliced
- 2 tbsp vermouth
- ½ tsp garlic powder
- 1 tbsp olive oil
- 2 tsp herbs
- 1 tbsp duck fat, softened

Directions:
1. In a bowl, mix the duck fat, garlic powder, and herbs. Rub the mushrooms with the mixture and place them in a baking tray. Drizzle with vermouth and cook in your for 15 minutes on Bake function at 350 F. Serve.

375. Cheese And Bean Enchiladas

Servings: x
Cooking Time: x
Ingredients:
- A pinch of salt or to taste
- A few red chili flakes to sprinkle
- 1 tsp. of oregano
- 2 tbsp. oil
- 2 tsp. chopped garlic
- 2 onions chopped finely
- 2 capsicums chopped finely
- 2 cups of readymade baked beans
- Flour tortillas (as many as required)
- 4 tbsp. of olive oil
- A pinch of salt
- 1 tsp. oregano
- ½ tsp. pepper
- 1 ½ tsp. red chili flakes or to taste
- 1 tbsp. of finely chopped jalapenos
- 1 cup grated pizza cheese (mix mozzarella and cheddar cheeses)
- 1 ½ tsp. of garlic that has been chopped
- 1 ½ cups of readymade tomato puree
- 3 medium tomatoes. Puree them in a mixer
- 1 tsp. of sugar
- A few drops of Tabasco sauce
- 1 cup crumbled or roughly mashed cottage cheese (cottage cheese)
- 1 cup grated cheddar cheese

Directions:
1. Prepare the flour tortillas. Now move on to making the red sauce. In a pan, pour around 2 tbsp. of oil and heat. Add some garlic. Add

the rest of the ingredients mentioned under the heading "For the sauce".

2. Keep stirring. Cook until the sauce reduces and becomes thick. For the filling, heat one tbsp. of oil in another pan. Add onions and garlic and cook until the onions are caramelized or attain a golden-brown color. Add the rest of the ingredients required for the filling and cook for two to three minutes.

3. Take the pan off the flame and grate some cheese over the sauce. Mix it well and let it sit for a while. Let us start assembling the dish. Take a tortilla and spread some of the sauce on the surface. Now place the filling at the center in a line. Roll up the tortilla carefully. Do the same for all the tortillas. Now place all the tortillas in a tray and sprinkle them with grated cheese. Cover this with an aluminum foil. Pre heat the oven at 160° C for 4-5 minutes. Open the basket and place the tray inside.

4. Keep the fryer at the same temperature for another 15 minutes. Turn the tortillas over in between to get a uniform cook.

376.Parmesan Breaded Zucchini Chips

Servings: 5
Cooking Time: 20 Minutes
Ingredients:
- For the zucchini chips:
- 2 medium zucchini
- 2 eggs
- ⅓ cup bread crumbs
- ⅓ cup grated Parmesan cheese
- Salt
- Pepper
- Cooking oil
- For the lemon aioli:
- ½ cup mayonnaise
- ½ tablespoon olive oil
- Juice of ½ lemon
- 1 teaspoon minced garlic
- Salt
- Pepper

Directions:
1. Preparing the Ingredients. To make the zucchini chips:
2. Slice the zucchini into thin chips (about ⅛ inch thick) using a knife or mandoline.
3. In a small bowl, beat the eggs. In another small bowl, combine the bread crumbs, Parmesan cheese, and salt and pepper to taste.
4. Spray the Oven rack/basket with cooking oil.
5. Dip the zucchini slices one at a time in the eggs and then the bread crumb mixture. You can also sprinkle the bread crumbs onto the zucchini slices with a spoon.

6. Place the zucchini chips in the Oven rack/basket, but do not stack. Place the Rack on the middle-shelf of the air fryer oven.
7. Air Frying. Cook in batches. Spray the chips with cooking oil from a distance (otherwise, the breading may fly off). Cook for 10 minutes.
8. Remove the cooked zucchini chips from the air fryer oven, then repeat step 5 with the remaining zucchini.
9. To make the lemon aioli:
10. While the zucchini is cooking, combine the mayonnaise, olive oil, lemon juice, and garlic in a small bowl, adding salt and pepper to taste. Mix well until fully combined.
11. Cool the zucchini and serve alongside the aioli.
- **Nutrition Info:** CALORIES: 192; FAT: 13G; PROTEIN: 6

377.Cauliflower French Cuisine Galette

Servings:x
Cooking Time:x
Ingredients:
- 3 tsp. ginger finely chopped
- 1-2 tbsp. fresh coriander leaves
- 2 or 3 green chilies finely chopped
- 1 ½ tbsp. lemon juice
- Salt and pepper to taste
- 2 tbsp. garam masala
- 2 cups cauliflower
- 1 ½ cup coarsely crushed peanuts

Directions:
1. Mix the ingredients in a clean bowl.
2. Mold this mixture into round and flat French Cuisine Galettes.
3. Wet the French Cuisine Galettes slightly with water. Coat each French Cuisine Galette with the crushed peanuts.
4. Pre heat the oven at 160 degrees Fahrenheit for 5 minutes. Place the French Cuisine Galettes in the fry basket and let them cook for another 25 minutes at the same temperature. Keep rolling them over to get a uniform cook. Serve either with mint sauce or ketchup.

378.Snake Gourd French Cuisine Galette

Servings:x
Cooking Time:x
Ingredients:
- 1-2 tbsp. fresh coriander leaves
- 2 or 3 green chilies finely chopped
- 1 ½ tbsp. lemon juice
- Salt and pepper to taste
- 2 tbsp. garam masala
- 1 cup sliced snake gourd

- 1 ½ cup coarsely crushed peanuts
- 3 tsp. ginger finely chopped

Directions:
1. Mix the ingredients in a clean bowl.
2. Mold this mixture into round and flat French Cuisine Galettes.
3. Wet the French Cuisine Galettes slightly with water. Coat each French Cuisine Galette with the crushed peanuts.
4. Pre heat the oven at 160 degrees Fahrenheit for 5 minutes. Place the French Cuisine Galettes in the fry basket and let them cook for another 25 minutes at the same temperature. Keep rolling them over to get a uniform cook. Serve either with mint sauce or ketchup.

379.Chickpea & Carrot Balls

Servings: 3
Cooking Time: 25 Minutes
Ingredients:
- 2 tbsp olive oil
- 2 tbsp soy sauce
- 1 tbsp flax meal
- 2 cups cooked chickpeas
- ½ cup sweet onions
- ½ cup grated carrots
- ½ cup roasted cashews
- Juice of 1 lemon
- ½ tsp turmeric
- 1 tsp cumin
- 1 tsp garlic powder
- 1 cup rolled oats

Directions:
1. Combine the olive oil, onions, and carrots into the Air Fryer baking pan and cook them on Air Fry function for 6 minutes at 350 F. Ground the oats and cashews in a food processor. Place in a large bowl. Mix in the chickpeas, lemon juice, and soy sauce.
2. Add onions and carrots to the bowl with chickpeas. Stir in the remaining ingredients; mix until fully incorporated. Make meatballs out of the mixture. Increase the temperature to 370 F and cook for 12 minutes.

380.Tortellini With Veggies And Parmesan

Servings:4
Cooking Time: 16 Minutes
Ingredients:
- 8 ounces (227 g) sugar snap peas, trimmed
- ½ pound (227 g) asparagus, trimmed and cut into 1-inch pieces
- 2 teaspoons kosher salt or 1 teaspoon fine salt, divided
- 1 tablespoon extra-virgin olive oil
- 1½ cups water

- 1 (20-ounce / 340-g) package frozen cheese tortellini
- 2 garlic cloves, minced
- 1 cup heavy (whipping) cream
- 1 cup cherry tomatoes, halved
- ½ cup grated Parmesan cheese
- ¼ cup chopped fresh parsley or basil
- Add the peas and asparagus to a large bowl. Add ½ teaspoon of kosher salt and the olive oil and toss until well coated. Place the veggies in the baking pan.

Directions:
1. Slide the baking pan into Rack Position 1, select Convection Bake, set the temperature to 450ºF (235ºC), and set the time for 4 minutes.
2. Meanwhile, dissolve 1 teaspoon of kosher salt in the water.
3. Once cooking is complete, remove the pan from the oven and place the tortellini in the pan. Pour the salted water over the tortellini. Put the pan back to the oven.
4. Slide the baking pan into Rack Position 1, select Convection Bake, set temperature to 450ºF (235ºC), and set time for 7 minutes.
5. Meantime, stir together the garlic, heavy cream, and remaining ½ teaspoon of kosher salt in a small bowl.
6. Once cooking is complete, remove the pan from the oven. Blot off any remaining water with a paper towel. Gently stir the ingredients. Drizzle the cream over and top with the tomatoes.
7. Slide the baking pan into Rack Position 2, select Roast, set the temperature to 375ºF (190ºC), and set the time for 5 minutes.
8. After 4 minutes, remove from the oven.
9. Add the Parmesan cheese and stir until the cheese is melted
10. Serve topped with the parsley.

381.Zucchini Parmesan Chips

Servings: 10
Cooking Time: 8 Minutes
Ingredients:
- ½ tsp. paprika
- ½ C. grated parmesan cheese
- ½ C. Italian breadcrumbs
- 1 lightly beaten egg
- 2 thinly sliced zucchinis

Directions:
1. Preparing the Ingredients. Use a very sharp knife or mandolin slicer to slice zucchini as thinly as you can. Pat off extra moisture.
2. Beat egg with a pinch of pepper and salt and a bit of water.
3. Combine paprika, cheese, and breadcrumbs in a bowl.

4. Dip slices of zucchini into the egg mixture and then into breadcrumb mixture. Press gently to coat.
5. Air Frying. With olive oil cooking spray, mist coated zucchini slices. Place into your air fryer oven in a single layer. Set temperature to 350°F, and set time to 8 minutes.
6. Sprinkle with salt and serve with salsa.
- **Nutrition Info:** CALORIES: 211; FAT: 16G; PROTEIN:8G; SUGAR:0G

382.Colorful Vegetarian Delight

Servings: 2
Cooking Time: 25 Minutes
Ingredients:
- 1 parsnip, sliced in a 2-inch thickness
- 1 cup chopped butternut squash
- 2 small red onions, cut in wedges
- 1 cup chopped celery
- 1 tbsp chopped fresh thyme
- Salt and black pepper to taste
- 2 tsp olive oil

Directions:
1. Preheat on Air Fry function to 380 F. In a bowl, add turnip, squash, red onions, celery, thyme, pepper, salt, and olive oil; mix well. Add the veggies to the basket and fit in the baking tray; cook for 16 minutes, tossing once halfway through. Serve.

383.Potato Fried Baked Pastry

Servings:x
Cooking Time:x
Ingredients:
- 1 tsp. powdered ginger
- 1 or 2 green chilies that are finely chopped or mashed
- ½ tsp. cumin
- 1 tsp. coarsely crushed coriander
- 1 dry red chili broken into pieces
- A small amount of salt (to taste)
- 2 tbsp. unsalted butter
- 1 ½ cup all-purpose flour
- A pinch of salt to taste
- Add as much water as required to make the dough stiff and firm
- 2-3 big potatoes boiled and mashed
- ¼ cup boiled peas
- ½ tsp. dried mango powder
- ½ tsp. red chili power.
- 1-2 tbsp. coriander.

Directions:
1. Mix the dough for the outer covering and make it stiff and smooth. Leave it to rest in a container while making the filling. Cook the ingredients in a pan and stir them well to make a thick paste. Roll the paste out.

2. Roll the dough into balls and flatten them. Cut them in halves and add the filling. Use water to help you fold the edges to create the shape of a cone. Pre-heat the oven for around 5 to 6 minutes at 300 Fahrenheit.
3. Place all the samosas in the fry basket and close the basket properly. Keep the oven at 200 degrees for another 20 to 25 minutes. Around the halfway point, open the basket and turn the samosas over for uniform cooking. After this, fry at 250 degrees for around 10 minutes in order to give them the desired golden-brown color. Serve hot. Recommended sides are tamarind or mint sauce.

384.Parsley Hearty Carrots

Servings: 3
Cooking Time: 25 Minutes
Ingredients:
- 2 tsp olive oil
- 2 shallots, chopped
- 3 carrots, sliced
- Salt to taste
- ¼ cup yogurt
- 2 garlic cloves, minced
- 3 tbsp parsley, chopped

Directions:
1. In a baking dish, mix olive oil, carrots, salt, garlic, shallots, parsley, and yogurt.
2. Place the dish in your and cook for 15 minutes on Bake function at 370 F. Serve with garlic mayo.

385.Mixed Vegetable Pancakes

Servings:x
Cooking Time:x
Ingredients:
- 2 cups shredded vegetables
- Salt and Pepper to taste
- 3 tbsp. Butter
- 1 ½ cups almond flour
- 3 eggs
- 2 tsp. dried basil
- 2 tsp. dried parsley

Directions:
1. Preheat the air fryer to 250 Fahrenheit.
2. In a small bowl, mix the ingredients together. Ensure that the mixture is smooth and well balanced.
3. Take a pancake mold and grease it with butter. Add the batter to the mold and place it in the air fryer basket.
4. Cook till both the sides of the pancake have browned on both sides and serve with maple syrup.

386.Broccoli Momo's Recipe

Servings:x

Cooking Time:x
Ingredients:
- 2 tbsp. oil
- 2 tsp. ginger-garlic paste
- 2 tsp. soya sauce
- 2 tsp. vinegar
- 1 ½ cup all-purpose flour
- ½ tsp. salt
- 5 tbsp. water
- 2 cups grated broccoli

Directions:
1. Squeeze the dough and cover it with plastic wrap and set aside. Next, cook the ingredients for the filling and try to ensure that the broccoli is covered well with the sauce.
2. Roll the dough and cut it into a square. Place the filling in the center. Now, wrap the dough to cover the filling and pinch the edges together.
3. Pre heat the oven at 200° F for 5 minutes. Place the gnocchi's in the fry basket and close it. Let them cook at the same temperature for another 20 minutes. Recommended sides are chili sauce or ketchup.

387. Jalapeño Cheese Balls

Servings: 12
Cooking Time: 8 Minutes
Ingredients:
- 4 ounces cream cheese
- ⅓ cup shredded mozzarella cheese
- ⅓ cup shredded Cheddar cheese
- 2 jalapeños, finely chopped
- ½ cup bread crumbs
- 2 eggs
- ½ cup all-purpose flour
- Salt
- Pepper
- Cooking oil

Directions:
1. Preparing the Ingredients. In a medium bowl, combine the cream cheese, mozzarella, Cheddar, and jalapeños. Mix well.
2. Form the cheese mixture into balls about an inch thick. Using a small ice cream scoop works well.
3. Arrange the cheese balls on a sheet pan and place in the freezer for 15 minutes. This will help the cheese balls maintain their shape while frying.
4. Spray the Oven rack/basket with cooking oil. Place the bread crumbs in a small bowl. In another small bowl, beat the eggs. In a third small bowl, combine the flour with salt and pepper to taste, and mix well. Remove the cheese balls from the freezer.

Dip the cheese balls in the flour, then the eggs, and then the bread crumbs.
5. Air Frying. Place the cheese balls in the Oven rack/basket. Spray with cooking oil. Place the Rack on the middle-shelf of the air fryer oven. Cook for 8 minutes.
6. Open the air fryer oven and flip the cheese balls. I recommend flipping them instead of shaking, so the balls maintain their form. Cook an additional 4 minutes. Cool before serving.
- **Nutrition Info:** CALORIES: 96; FAT: 6G; PROTEIN:4G; SUGAR:

388. Chili Veggie Skewers

Servings: 4
Cooking Time: 20 Minutes
Ingredients:
- 2 tbsp cornflour
- 1 cup canned white beans, drained
- ⅓ cup grated carrots
- 2 boiled and mashed potatoes
- ¼ cup chopped fresh mint leaves
- ½ tsp garam masala powder
- ½ cup paneer
- 1 green chili
- 1-inch piece of fresh ginger
- 3 garlic cloves
- Salt to taste

Directions:
1. Preheat on Air Fry function to 390 F. Place the beans, carrots, garlic, ginger, chili, paneer, and mint in a food processor; process until smooth. Transfer to a bowl. Add in the mashed potatoes, cornflour, salt, and garam masala powder and mix until fully incorporated.
2. Divide the mixture into 12 equal pieces. Shape each of the pieces around a skewer. Cook in your for 10 minutes, turning once. Serve.

389. Roasted Vegetables With Basil

Servings:2
Cooking Time: 20 Minutes
Ingredients:
- 1 small eggplant, halved and sliced
- 1 yellow bell pepper, cut into thick strips
- 1 red bell pepper, cut into thick strips
- 2 garlic cloves, quartered
- 1 red onion, sliced
- 1 tablespoon extra-virgin olive oil
- Salt and freshly ground black pepper, to taste
- ½ cup chopped fresh basil, for garnish
- Cooking spray

Directions:
1. Grease the baking pan with cooking spray.

2. Place the eggplant, bell peppers, garlic, and red onion in the greased baking pan. Drizzle with the olive oil and toss to coat well. Spritz any uncoated surfaces with cooking spray.
3. Slide the baking pan into Rack Position 1, select Convection Bake, set temperature to 350ºF (180ºC), and set time to 20 minutes.
4. Flip the vegetables halfway through the cooking time.
5. When done, remove from the oven and sprinkle with salt and pepper.
6. Sprinkle the basil on top for garnish and serve.

390.Roasted Butternut Squash With Maple Syrup

Servings:4
Cooking Time: 30 Minutes
Ingredients:
- 1 lb butternut squash
- 1 tsp dried rosemary
- 2 tbsp maple syrup
- Salt to taste

Directions:
1. Place the squash on a cutting board and peel. Cut in half and remove the seeds and pulp. Slice into wedges and season with salt. Spray with cooking spray and sprinkle with rosemary.
2. Preheat on AirFry function to 350 F. Transfer the wedges to the greased basket without overlapping. Press Start and cook for 20 minutes. Serve drizzled with maple syrup.

391.Vegetable And Cheese Stuffed Tomatoes

Servings:4
Cooking Time: 18 Minutes
Ingredients:
- 4 medium beefsteak tomatoes, rinsed
- ½ cup grated carrot
- 1 medium onion, chopped
- 1 garlic clove, minced
- 2 teaspoons olive oil
- 2 cups fresh baby spinach
- ¼ cup crumbled low-sodium feta cheese
- ½ teaspoon dried basil

Directions:
1. On your cutting board, cut a thin slice off the top of each tomato. Scoop out a ¼- to ½-inch-thick tomato pulp and place the tomatoes upside down on paper towels to drain. Set aside.
2. Stir together the carrot, onion, garlic, and olive oil in the baking pan.

3. Slide the baking pan into Rack Position 1, select Convection Bake, set temperature to 350ºF (180ºC) and set time to 5 minutes.
4. Stir the vegetables halfway through.
5. When cooking is complete, the carrot should be crisp-tender.
6. Remove from the oven and stir in the spinach, feta cheese, and basil.
7. Spoon ¼ of the vegetable mixture into each tomato and transfer the stuffed tomatoes to the oven. Set time to 13 minutes.
8. When cooking is complete, the filling should be hot and the tomatoes should be lightly caramelized.
9. Let the tomatoes cool for 5 minutes and serve.

392.Garlicky Veggie Bake

Servings: 3
Cooking Time: 25 Minutes
Ingredients:
- 3 turnips, sliced
- 1 large red onion, cut into rings
- 1 large zucchini, sliced
- Salt and black pepper to taste
- 2 cloves garlic, crushed
- 1 bay leaf, cut in 6 pieces
- 1 tbsp olive oil

Directions:
1. Place the turnips, onion, and zucchini in a bowl. Toss with olive oil, salt, and pepper.
2. Preheat on Air Fry function to 380 F. Place the veggies into a baking pan. Slip the bay leaves in the different parts of the slices and tuck the garlic cloves in between the slices. Cook for 15 minutes. Serve warm with as a side to a meat dish or salad.

393.Cayenne Spicy Green Beans

Servings: 4
Cooking Time: 20 Minutes
Ingredients:
- 1 cup panko breadcrumbs
- 2 whole eggs, beaten
- ½ cup Parmesan cheese, grated
- ½ cup flour
- 1 tsp cayenne pepper
- 1 ½ pounds green beans
- Salt to taste

Directions:
1. In a bowl, mix panko breadcrumbs, Parmesan cheese, cayenne pepper, salt, and pepper. Roll the green beans in flour and dip in eggs. Dredge beans in the parmesan-panko mix. Place the prepared beans in the greased cooking basket and fit in the baking tray; cook for 15 minutes on Air Fry function at 350 F, shaking once. Serve and enjoy!

394.Cottage Cheese Patties

Servings:x
Cooking Time:x
Ingredients:
- 1 tbsp. fresh coriander leaves
- ¼ tsp. red chili powder
- ¼ tsp. cumin powder
- 1 cup grated cottage cheese
- A pinch of salt to taste
- ¼ tsp. ginger finely chopped
- 1 green chili finely chopped
- 1 tsp. lemon juice

Directions:
1. Mix the ingredients together and ensure that the flavors are right. You will now make round patties with the mixture and roll them out well.
2. Pre heat the oven at 250 Fahrenheit for 5 minutes. Open the basket of the Fryer and arrange the patties in the basket. Close it carefully. Keep the
3. fryer at 150 degrees for around 10 or 12 minutes. In between the cooking process, turn the patties over to get a uniform cook. Serve hot with mint sauce.

395.White Lentil French Cuisine Galette

Servings:x
Cooking Time:x
Ingredients:
- 1 ½ tbsp. lemon juice
- Salt and pepper to taste
- 2 cup white lentil soaked
- 3 tsp. ginger finely chopped
- 1-2 tbsp. fresh coriander leaves
- 2 or 3 green chilies finely chopped

Directions:
1. Wash the soaked lentils and mix it with the rest of the ingredients in a clean bowl.
2. Mold this mixture into round and flat French Cuisine Galettes.
3. Wet the French Cuisine Galettes slightly with water.
4. Pre heat the oven at 160 degrees Fahrenheit for 5 minutes. Place the French Cuisine Galettes in the fry basket and let them cook for another 25 minutes at the same temperature. Keep rolling them over to get a uniform cook. Serve either with mint sauce or ketchup.

396.Cottage Cheese Flat Cakes

Servings:x
Cooking Time:x
Ingredients:
- 2 or 3 green chilies finely chopped
- 1 ½ tbsp. lemon juice
- Salt and pepper to taste
- 2 tbsp. garam masala

- 2 cups sliced cottage cheese
- 3 tsp. ginger finely chopped
- 1-2 tbsp. fresh coriander leaves

Directions:
1. Mix the ingredients in a clean bowl and add water to it. Make sure that the paste is not too watery but is enough to apply on the cottage cheese slices.
2. Pre heat the oven at 160 degrees Fahrenheit for 5 minutes. Place the French Cuisine Galettes in the fry basket and let them cook for another 25 minutes at the same temperature. Keep rolling them over to get a uniform cook. Serve either with mint sauce or ketchup.

397.Rosemary Squash With Cheese

Servings: 2
Cooking Time: 20 Minutes
Ingredients:
- 1 pound (454 g) butternut squash, cut into wedges
- 2 tablespoons olive oil
- 1 tablespoon dried rosemary
- Salt, to salt
- 1 cup crumbled goat cheese
- 1 tablespoon maple syrup

Directions:
1. Toss the squash wedges with the olive oil, rosemary, and salt in a large bowl until well coated.
2. Transfer the squash wedges to the air fryer basket, spreading them out in as even a layer as possible.
3. Put the air fryer basket on the baking pan and slide into Rack Position 2, select Air Fry, set temperature to 350ºF (180ºC), and set time to 20 minutes.
4. After 10 minutes, remove from the oven and flip the squash. Return the pan to the oven and continue cooking for 10 minutes.
5. When cooking is complete, the squash should be golden brown. Remove from the oven. Sprinkle the goat cheese on top and serve drizzled with the maple syrup.

398.Mediterranean Baked Eggs With Spinach

Servings:2
Cooking Time: 10 Minutes
Ingredients:
- 2 tablespoons olive oil
- 4 eggs, whisked
- 5 ounces (142 g) fresh spinach, chopped
- 1 medium-sized tomato, chopped
- 1 teaspoon fresh lemon juice
- ½ teaspoon ground black pepper
- ½ teaspoon coarse salt

- ½ cup roughly chopped fresh basil leaves, for garnish

Directions:
1. Generously grease the baking pan with olive oil.
2. Stir together the remaining ingredients except the basil leaves in the greased baking pan until well incorporated.
3. Slide the baking pan into Rack Position 1, select Convection Bake, set temperature to 280ºF (137ºC), and set time to 10 minutes.
4. When cooking is complete, the eggs should be completely set and the vegetables should be tender. Remove from the oven and serve garnished with the fresh basil leaves.

399.Cayenne Tahini Kale

Servings:2 To 4
Cooking Time: 15 Minutes
Ingredients:
- Dressing:
- ¼ cup tahini
- ¼ cup fresh lemon juice
- 2 tablespoons olive oil
- 1 teaspoon sesame seeds
- ½ teaspoon garlic powder
- ¼ teaspoon cayenne pepper
- Kale:
- 4 cups packed torn kale leaves (stems and ribs removed and leaves torn into palm-size pieces)
- Kosher salt and freshly ground black pepper, to taste

Directions:
1. Make the dressing: Whisk together the tahini, lemon juice, olive oil, sesame seeds, garlic powder, and cayenne pepper in a large bowl until well mixed.
2. Add the kale and massage the dressing thoroughly all over the leaves. Sprinkle the salt and pepper to season.
3. Place the kale in the air fryer basket in a single layer.
4. Put the air fryer basket on the baking pan and slide into Rack Position 2, select Air Fry, set temperature to 350ºF (180ºC), and set time to 15 minutes.
5. When cooking is complete, the leaves should be slightly wilted and crispy. Remove from the oven and serve on a plate.

SNACKS AND DESSERTS RECIPES

400.Almond Blueberry Bars

Servings: 4
Cooking Time: 50 Minutes
Ingredients:
- 1/4 cup blueberries
- 3 tbsp coconut oil
- 2 tbsp coconut flour
- 1/2 cup almond flour
- 3 tbsp water
- 1 tbsp chia seeds
- 1 tsp vanilla
- 1 tsp fresh lemon juice
- 2 tbsp erythritol
- 1/4 cup almonds, sliced
- 1/4 cup coconut flakes

Directions:
1. Fit the oven with the rack in position
2. Line baking dish with parchment paper and set aside.
3. In a small bowl, mix together water and chia seeds. Set aside.
4. In a bowl, combine together all ingredients. Add chia mixture and stir well.
5. Pour mixture into the prepared baking dish and spread evenly.
6. Set to bake at 300 F for 55 minutes. After 5 minutes place the baking dish in the preheated oven.
7. Slice and serve.
- **Nutrition Info:** Calories 208 Fat 18.2 g Carbohydrates 9.1 g Sugar 2.3 g Protein 3.6 g Cholesterol 0 mg

401.Tofu Steaks

Servings: 4
Cooking Time: 35 Minutes
Ingredients:
- 1 package tofu, press and remove excess liquid
- 2 tbsp lemon zest
- 3 garlic cloves, minced
- 1/4 cup olive oil
- 1/4 tsp dried thyme
- 1/4 cup lemon juice
- Pepper
- Salt

Directions:
1. Fit the oven with the rack in position 2.
2. Cut tofu into eight pieces.
3. In a bowl, mix together olive oil, thyme, lemon juice, lemon zest, garlic, pepper, and salt.
4. Add tofu into the bowl and coat well and place it in the refrigerator overnight.
5. Place marinated tofu in an air fryer basket then places an air fryer basket in the baking pan.

6. Place a baking pan on the oven rack. Set to air fry at 350 F for 35 minutes.
7. Serve and enjoy.
- **Nutrition Info:** Calories 139 Fat 14.1 g Carbohydrates 2.3 g Sugar 0.7 g Protein 2.9 g Cholesterol 0 mg

402.Easy Almond Butter Pumpkin Spice Cookies

Servings: 6
Cooking Time: 18 Minutes
Ingredients:
- 1/4 tsp pumpkin pie spice
- 1 tsp liquid Stevie
- 6 oz almond butter
- 1/3 cup pumpkin puree

Directions:
1. Fit the oven with the rack in position
2. Add all ingredients into the food processor and process until just combined.
3. Drop spoonfuls of mixture onto the parchment-lined baking pan.
4. Set to bake at 350 F for 23 minutes. After 5 minutes place the baking pan in the preheated oven.
5. Serve and enjoy.
- **Nutrition Info:** Calories 85 Fat 7 g Carbohydrates 3 g Sugar 1 g Protein 3 g Cholesterol 0 mg

403.Bbq Pulled Mushrooms

Servings: 2
Cooking Time: 15 Minutes
Ingredients:
- 4 large portobello mushrooms
- ½ cup low-carb, sugar-free barbecue sauce
- 1 tbsp. salted butter; melted.
- 1 tsp. paprika
- ¼ tsp. onion powder.
- ¼ tsp. ground black pepper
- 1 tsp. chili powder

Directions:
1. Remove stem and scoop out the underside of each mushroom. Brush the caps with butter and sprinkle with pepper, chili powder, paprika and onion powder.
2. Place mushrooms into the air fryer basket. Adjust the temperature to 400 Degrees F and set the timer for 8 minutes.
3. When the timer beeps, remove mushrooms from the basket and place on a cutting board or work surface. Using two forks, gently pull the mushrooms apart, creating strands.
4. Place mushroom strands into a 4-cup round baking dish with barbecue sauce. Place dish into the air fryer basket.

5. Adjust the temperature to 350 Degrees F and set the timer for 4 minutes. Stir halfway through the cooking time. Serve warm.
- **Nutrition Info:** Calories: 108; Protein: 3.3g; Fiber: 2.7g; Fat: 5.9g; Carbs: 10.9g

404.Nan Khatam

Servings:x
Cooking Time:x
Ingredients:
- 1 tbsp. Unsalted Butter
- 1 tsp. baking powder
- 1 tsp. baking soda
- 1 tsp. cardamom powder
- 1 ½ cup all-purpose flour
- 1 cup Gram flour
- 1 cup +3 tbsp. icing sugar

Directions:
1. Create a crumbly mixture using the ingredients and make small balls of the mixture and flattening them on a prepared baking tray.
2. Preheat the fryer to 300 Fahrenheit for five minutes. Place the baking tray in the basket and reduce the temperature to 250 Fahrenheit. Cook both sides of the ball for five minutes to ensure that they are cooked uniformly. Once the nan khatam has cooled, store them in an airtight container.

405.Monkey Bread

Servings: 6
Cooking Time: 15 Minutes
Ingredients:
- ½ cup blanched finely ground almond flour.
- 1 oz. full-fat cream cheese; softened.
- 1 large egg.
- ¼ cup heavy whipping cream.
- ½ cup low-carb vanilla protein powder
- ¾ cup granular erythritol, divided
- 8 tbsp. salted butter; melted and divided
- ½ tsp. vanilla extract.
- ½ tsp. baking powder

Directions:
1. Take a large bowl, combine almond flour, protein powder, ½ cup erythritol, baking powder, 5 tbsp. butter, cream cheese and egg. A soft, sticky dough will form.
2. Place the dough in the freezer for 20 minutes. It will be firm enough to roll into balls. Wet your hands with warm water and roll into twelve balls. Place the balls into a 6-inch round baking dish
3. In a medium skillet over medium heat, melt remaining butter with remaining erythritol. Lower the heat and continue stirring until mixture turns golden, then add cream and vanilla. Remove from heat and allow it to

thicken for a few minutes while you continue to stir
4. While the mixture cools, place baking dish into the air fryer basket. Adjust the temperature to 320 Degrees F and set the timer for 6 minutes
5. When the timer beeps, flip the monkey bread over onto a plate and slide it back into the baking pan. Cook an additional 4 minutes until all the tops are brown.
6. Pour the caramel sauce over the monkey bread and cook an additional 2 minutes.
7. Let cool completely before serving.
- **Nutrition Info:** Calories: 322; Protein: 20.4g; Fiber: 1.7g; Fat: 24.5g; Carbs: 33.7g

406.Orange And Anise Cake

Servings:6
Cooking Time: 20 Minutes
Ingredients:
- 1 stick butter, at room temperature
- 5 tablespoons liquid monk fruit
- 2 eggs plus 1 egg yolk, beaten
- $1/3$ cup hazelnuts, roughly chopped
- 3 tablespoons sugar-free orange marmalade
- 6 ounces (170 g) unbleached almond flour
- 1 teaspoon baking soda
- ½ teaspoon baking powder
- ½ teaspoon ground cinnamon
- ½ teaspoon ground allspice
- ½ ground anise seed
- Cooking spray

Directions:
1. Lightly spritz the baking pan with cooking spray.
2. In a mixing bowl, whisk the butter and liquid monk fruit until the mixture is pale and smooth. Mix in the beaten eggs, hazelnuts, and marmalade and whisk again until well incorporated.
3. Add the almond flour, baking soda, baking powder, cinnamon, allspice, anise seed and stir to mix well.
4. Scrape the batter into the prepared baking pan.
5. Slide the baking pan into Rack Position 1, select Convection Bake, set temperature to 310ºF (154ºC), and set time to 20 minutes.
6. When cooking is complete, the top of the cake should spring back when gently pressed with your fingers.
7. Transfer to a wire rack and let the cake cool to room temperature. Serve immediately.

407.Cuban Sandwiches

Servings: 4 Sandwiches
Cooking Time: 8 Minutes
Ingredients:
- 8 slices ciabatta bread, about ¼-inch thick

116

- Cooking spray
- 1 tablespoon brown mustard
- Toppings:
- 6 to 8 ounces (170 to 227 g) thinly sliced leftover roast pork
- 4 ounces (113 g) thinly sliced deli turkey
- $^1/_3$ cup bread and butter pickle slices
- 2 to 3 ounces (57 to 85 g) Pepper Jack cheese slices

Directions:
1. On a clean work surface, spray one side of each slice of bread with cooking spray. Spread the other side of each slice of bread evenly with brown mustard.
2. Top 4 of the bread slices with the roast pork, turkey, pickle slices, cheese, and finish with remaining bread slices. Transfer to the air fryer basket.
3. Put the air fryer basket on the baking pan and slide into Rack Position 2, select Air Fry, set temperature to 390ºF (199ºC), and set time to 8 minutes.
4. When cooking is complete, remove from the oven. Cool for 5 minutes and serve warm.

408.Bacon Cheese Jalapeno Poppers

Servings: 5
Cooking Time: 5 Minutes
Ingredients:
- 10 fresh jalapeno peppers, cut in half and remove seeds
- 1/4 cup cheddar cheese, shredded
- 5 oz cream cheese, softened
- ¼ tsp paprika
- 2 bacon slices, cooked and crumbled

Directions:
1. Fit the oven with the rack in position 2.
2. In a bowl, mix bacon, cream cheese, paprika and cheddar cheese.
3. Stuff cheese mixture into each jalapeno.
4. Place stuffed jalapeno halved in air fryer basket then place air fryer basket in baking pan.
5. Place a baking pan on the oven rack. Set to air fry at 370 F for 5 minutes.
6. Serve and enjoy.
- **Nutrition Info:** Calories 176 Fat 15.7 g Carbohydrates 3.2 g Sugar 1 g Protein 6.2 g Cholesterol 47 mg

409.Paprika Deviled Eggs

Servings:12
Cooking Time: 16 Minutes
Ingredients:
- 3 cups ice
- 12 large eggs
- ½ cup mayonnaise
- 10 hamburger dill pickle chips, diced
- ¼ cup diced onion

- 2 teaspoons salt
- 2 teaspoons yellow mustard
- 1 teaspoon freshly ground black pepper
- ½ teaspoon paprika

Directions:
1. Put the ice in a large bowl and set aside. Carefully place the eggs in the baking pan.
2. Slide the baking pan into Rack Position 1, select Convection Bake, set temperature to 250ºF (121ºC), and set time to 16 minutes.
3. When cooking is complete, transfer the eggs to the large bowl of ice to cool.
4. When cool enough to handle, peel the eggs. Slice them in half lengthwise and scoop out yolks into a small bowl. Stir in the mayonnaise, pickles, onion, salt, mustard, and pepper. Mash the mixture with a fork until well combined.
5. Fill each egg white half with 1 to 2 teaspoons of the egg yolk mixture.
6. Sprinkle the paprika on top and serve immediately.

410.Vanilla And Oats Pudding

Servings:x
Cooking Time:x
Ingredients:
- 2 tbsp. custard powder
- 3 tbsp. powdered sugar
- 3 tbsp. unsalted butter
- 2 cups vanilla powder
- 2 cups milk
- 1 cup oats

Directions:
1. Boil the milk and the sugar in a pan and add the custard powder followed by the vanilla powder followed by the oats and stir till you get a thick mixture.
2. Preheat the fryer to 300 Fahrenheit for five minutes. Place the dish in the basket and reduce the temperature to 250 Fahrenheit. Cook for ten minutes and set aside to cool.

411.Carrot Chips

Servings:4
Cooking Time: 10 Minutes
Ingredients:
- 4 to 5 medium carrots, trimmed and thinly sliced
- 1 tablespoon olive oil, plus more for greasing
- 1 teaspoon seasoned salt

Directions:
1. Toss the carrot slices with 1 tablespoon of olive oil and salt in a medium bowl until thoroughly coated.
2. Grease the air fryer basket with the olive oil. Place the carrot slices in the greased pan.

3. Put the air fryer basket on the baking pan and slide into Rack Position 2, select Air Fry, set temperature to 390ºF (199ºC), and set time to 10 minutes.
4. Stir the carrot slices halfway through the cooking time.
5. When cooking is complete, the chips should be crisp-tender. Remove from the oven and allow to cool for 5 minutes before serving.

412.Moist Chocolate Brownies

Servings: 16
Cooking Time: 20 Minutes
Ingredients:
- 1 1/3 cups all-purpose flour
- 1/2 tsp baking powder
- 1/3 cup cocoa powder
- 1 cup of sugar
- 1/2 tsp vanilla
- 1/2 cup vegetable oil
- 1/2 cup water
- 1/2 tsp salt

Directions:
1. Fit the oven with the rack in position
2. In a large mixing bowl, mix together flour, baking powder, cocoa powder, sugar, and salt.
3. In a small bowl, whisk together oil, water, and vanilla.
4. Pour oil mixture into the flour mixture and mix until well combined.
5. Pour batter into the greased baking dish.
6. Set to bake at 350 F for 25 minutes. After 5 minutes place the baking dish in the preheated oven.
7. Slice and serve.
- **Nutrition Info:** Calories 150 Fat 7.1 g Carbohydrates 21.5 g Sugar 12.6 g Protein 1.4 g Cholesterol 0 mg

413.Garlic Cauliflower Florets

Servings: 4
Cooking Time: 20 Minutes
Ingredients:
- 5 cups cauliflower florets
- 6 garlic cloves, chopped
- 4 tablespoons olive oil
- 1/2 tsp cumin powder
- 1/2 tsp salt

Directions:
1. Fit the oven with the rack in position 2.
2. Add all ingredients into the large bowl and toss well.
3. Add cauliflower florets in air fryer basket then place air fryer basket in baking pan.
4. Place a baking pan on the oven rack. Set to air fry at 400 F for 20 minutes.
5. Serve and enjoy.

- **Nutrition Info:** Calories 159 Fat 14.2 g Carbohydrates 8.2 g Sugar 3.1 g Protein 2.8 g Cholesterol 0 mg

414.Easy Bacon Jalapeno Poppers

Servings: 10
Cooking Time: 8 Minutes
Ingredients:
- 10 jalapeno peppers, cut in half and remove seeds
- 1/3 cup cream cheese, softened
- 1/4 tsp paprika
- 1/4 tsp chili powder
- 5 bacon strips, cut in half

Directions:
1. Fit the oven with the rack in position 2.
2. In a small bowl, mix cream cheese, paprika, chili powder, and bacon and stuff in each jalapeno half.
3. Place jalapeno half in the air fryer basket then place an air fryer basket in the baking pan.
4. Place a baking pan on the oven rack. Set to air fry at 370 F for 8 minutes.
5. Serve and enjoy.
- **Nutrition Info:** Calories 83 Fat 7.4 g Carbohydrates 1.3 g Sugar 0.5 g Protein 2.8 g Cholesterol 9 mg

415.Polenta Fries With Chili-lime Mayo

Servings:4
Cooking Time: 28 Minutes
Ingredients:
- Polenta Fries:
- 2 teaspoons vegetable or olive oil
- ¼ teaspoon paprika
- 1 pound (454 g) prepared polenta, cut into 3-inch × ½-inch strips
- Salt and freshly ground black pepper, to taste
- Chili-Lime Mayo:
- ½ cup mayonnaise
- 1 teaspoon chili powder
- 1 teaspoon chopped fresh cilantro
- ¼ teaspoon ground cumin
- Juice of ½ lime
- Salt and freshly ground black pepper, to taste

Directions:
1. Mix the oil and paprika in a bowl. Add the polenta strips and toss until evenly coated. Transfer the polenta strips to the air fryer basket.
2. Put the air fryer basket on the baking pan and slide into Rack Position 2, select Air Fry, set temperature to 400ºF (205ºC), and set time to 28 minutes.
3. Stir the polenta strips halfway through the cooking time.

4. Meanwhile, whisk together all the ingredients for the chili-lime mayo in a small bowl.
5. When cooking is complete, remove the polenta fries from the oven to a plate. Season as desired with salt and pepper. Serve alongside the chili-lime mayo as a dipping sauce.

416. Almond Flour Blackberry Muffins

Servings:8
Cooking Time: 12 Minutes
Ingredients:
- ½ cup fresh blackberries
- Dry Ingredients:
- 1½ cups almond flour
- 1 teaspoon baking powder
- ½ teaspoon baking soda
- ½ cup Swerve
- ¼ teaspoon kosher salt
- Wet Ingredients:
- 2 eggs
- ¼ cup coconut oil, melted
- ½ cup milk
- ½ teaspoon vanilla paste

Directions:
1. Line an 8-cup muffin tin with paper liners.
2. Thoroughly combine the almond flour, baking powder, baking soda, Swerve, and salt in a mixing bowl.
3. Whisk together the eggs, coconut oil, milk, and vanilla in a separate mixing bowl until smooth.
4. Add the wet mixture to the dry and fold in the blackberries. Stir with a spatula just until well incorporated.
5. Spoon the batter into the prepared muffin cups, filling each about three-quarters full.
6. Put the muffin tin into Rack Position 1, select Convection Bake, set temperature to 350ºF (180ºC), and set time to 12 minutes.
7. When done, the tops should be golden and a toothpick inserted in the middle should come out clean.
8. Allow the muffins to cool in the muffin tin for 10 minutes before removing and serving

417. Delicious Jalapeno Poppers

Servings: 10
Cooking Time: 7 Minutes
Ingredients:
- 10 jalapeno peppers, cut in half, remove seeds & membranes
- 1/2 cup cheddar cheese, shredded
- 4 oz cream cheese
- 1/4 tsp paprika
- 1 tsp ground cumin
- 1 tsp salt

Directions:

1. Fit the oven with the rack in position 2.
2. In a small bowl, mix together cream cheese, cheddar cheese, cumin, paprika, and salt.
3. Stuff cream cheese mixture into each jalapeno half.
4. Place stuffed jalapeno peppers in air fryer basket then place air fryer basket in baking pan.
5. Place a baking pan on the oven rack. Set to air fry at 350 F for 7 minutes.
6. Serve and enjoy.
- **Nutrition Info:** Calories 69 Fat 6.1 g Carbohydrates 1.5 g Sugar 0.5 g Protein 2.5 g Cholesterol 18 mg

418. Chocolate Tarts

Servings:x
Cooking Time:x
Ingredients:
- 1 tbsp. sliced cashew
- For Truffle filling:
- 1 ½ melted chocolate
- 1 cup fresh cream
- 3 tbsp. butter
- 1 ½ cup plain flour
- ½ cup cocoa powder
- 3 tbsp. unsalted butter
- 2 tbsp. powdered sugar
- 2 cups cold water

Directions:
1. In a large bowl, mix the flour, cocoa powder, butter and sugar with your Oregano Fingers. The mixture should resemble breadcrumbs. Squeeze the dough using the cold milk and wrap it and leave it to cool for ten minutes. Roll the dough out into the pie and prick the sides of the pie.
2. Mix the ingredients for the filling in a bowl. Make sure that it is a little thick. Add the filling to the pie and cover it with the second round.
3. Preheat the fryer to 300 Fahrenheit for five minutes. You will need to place the tin in the basket and cover it. When the pastry has turned golden brown, you will need to remove the tin and let it cool. Cut into slices and serve with a dollop of cream.

419. Simple Strawberry Cobbler

Servings: 4
Cooking Time: 25 Minutes
Ingredients:
- Butter, 2 tsps.
- Hulled strawberries, 1 ½ cup
- White sugar, 1 ½ tsps.
- Diced butter, 1 tbsp.
- Butter, 1 tbsp.
- All-purpose flour, ½ cup
- Heavy whipping cream, ¼ cup

- Cornstarch, 1 ½ tsps.
- White sugar, ¼ cup
- Water, ½ cup
- Salt, ¼ tsp.
- Baking powder, ¾ tsp.

Directions:
1. Lightly grease a baking pan of air fryer with cooking spray. Add water, cornstarch, and sugar. Cook for 10 minutes 390 °F or until hot and thick. Add strawberries and mix well. Dot tops with 1 tablespoon butter.
2. In a bowl, mix well salt, baking powder, sugar, and flour. Cut in 1 tablespoon and 2 teaspoons butter. Mix in cream. Spoon on top of berries.
3. Cook for 15 minutes at 390 °F, until tops are lightly browned.
4. Serve and enjoy.
- **Nutrition Info:** Calories: 255 Protein: 2.4g Fat: 13.0g Carbs: 32.0g

420.Vanilla-lemon Cupcakes With Lemon Glaze

Servings:6
Cooking Time: 30 Minutes
Ingredients:
- 1 cup flour
- ½ cup sugar
- 1 small egg
- 1 tsp lemon zest
- ¾ tsp baking powder
- ¼ tsp baking soda
- ½ tsp salt
- 2 tbsp vegetable oil
- ½ cup milk
- ½ tsp vanilla extract
- Glaze:
- ½ cup powdered sugar
- 2 tsp lemon juice

Directions:
1. Preheat on Bake function to 350 F. In a bowl, combine all dry muffin ingredients. In another bowl, whisk together the wet ingredients. Gently combine the two mixtures.
2. Divide the batter between 6 greased muffin tins. Place the tins in the oven and cook for 13 to 16 minutes. Whisk the powdered sugar with the lemon juice. Spread the glaze over the muffins.

421.Jalapeno Spinach Dip

Servings: 6
Cooking Time: 30 Minutes
Ingredients:
- 10 oz frozen spinach, thawed and drained
- 2 tsp jalapeno pepper, minced
- 1/2 cup cheddar cheese, shredded
- 8 oz cream cheese

- 1/2 cup onion, diced
- 2 tsp garlic, minced
- 1/2 cup mozzarella cheese, shredded
- 1/2 cup Monterey jack cheese, shredded
- 1/2 tsp salt

Directions:
1. Fit the oven with the rack in position
2. Add all ingredients into the mixing bowl and mix until well combined.
3. Pour mixture into the 1-quart casserole dish.
4. Set to bake at 350 F for 35 minutes. After 5 minutes place the casserole dish in the preheated oven.
5. Serve and enjoy.
- **Nutrition Info:** Calories 228 Fat 19.8 g Carbohydrates 4.2 g Sugar 0.8 g Protein 9.7 g Cholesterol 61 mg

422.Raspberry-coco Desert

Servings: 12
Cooking Time: 20 Minutes
Ingredients:
- Vanilla bean, 1 tsp.
- Pulsed raspberries, 1 cup
- Coconut milk, 1 cup
- Desiccated coconut, 3 cup
- Coconut oil, ¼ cup
- Erythritol powder, 1/3 cup

Directions:
1. Preheat the air fryer for 5 minutes.
2. Combine all ingredients in a mixing bowl.
3. Pour into a greased baking dish.
4. Bake in the air fryer for 20 minutes at 375 °F.
- **Nutrition Info:** Calories: 132 Carbs: 9.7g Fat: 9.7g Protein: 1.5g

423.Choco Cookies

Servings: 8
Cooking Time: 8 Minutes
Ingredients:
- 3 egg whites
- 3/4 cup cocoa powder, unsweetened
- 1 3/4 cup confectioner sugar
- 1 1/2 tsp vanilla

Directions:
1. Fit the oven with the rack in position
2. In a mixing bowl, whip egg whites until fluffy soft peaks. Slowly add in cocoa, sugar, and vanilla.
3. Drop teaspoonful onto parchment-lined baking pan into 32 small cookies.
4. Set to bake at 350 F for 8 minutes. After 5 minutes place the baking pan in the preheated oven.
5. Serve and enjoy.
- **Nutrition Info:** Calories 132 Fat 1.1 g Carbohydrates 31 g Sugar 0.3 g Protein 2 g Cholesterol 0 mg

424.Almond Cookies With Dark Chocolate

Servings:4
Cooking Time: 45 Minutes
Ingredients:
- 8 egg whites
- ½ tsp almond extract
- 1 ⅓ cups sugar
- ¼ tsp salt
- 2 tsp lemon juice
- 1 ½ tsp vanilla extract
- Melted dark chocolate to drizzle

Directions:
1. In a mixing bowl, add egg whites, salt, and lemon juice. Beat using an electric mixer until foamy.
2. Slowly add the sugar and continue beating until completely combined; add the almond and vanilla extracts. Beat until stiff and glossy peaks form.
3. Line a baking sheet with parchment paper. Fill a piping bag with the meringue mixture and pipe as many mounds on the baking sheet as you can leaving 2-inch spaces between each mound.
4. Place the baking sheet in the preheated oven and press Start. Bake at 250 F for 5 minutes on Bake function. Reduce the temperature to 220 F and bake for 15 more minutes.
5. Then, reduce the temperature to 190 F and cook for 15 minutes. Remove the baking sheet and let the meringues cool for 2 hours. Drizzle with dark chocolate and serve.

425.Coconut Butter Apple Bars

Servings: 8
Cooking Time: 45 Minutes
Ingredients:
- 1 tbsp ground flax seed
- 1/4 cup coconut butter, softened
- 1 cup pecans
- 1 cup of water
- 1/4 cup dried apples
- 1 1/2 tsp baking powder
- 1 1/2 tsp cinnamon
- 1 tsp vanilla
- 2 tbsp swerve

Directions:
1. Fit the oven with the rack in position
2. Add all ingredients into the blender and blend until smooth.
3. Pour blended mixture into the greased baking dish.
4. Set to bake at 350 F for 50 minutes. After 5 minutes place the baking dish in the preheated oven.
5. Slice and serve.

- **Nutrition Info:** Calories 161 Fat 15 g Carbohydrates 6 g Sugar 2 g Protein 2 g Cholesterol 0 mg

426.Air Fryer Chocolate Cake

Servings: 8-10
Cooking Time: 35 Minutes
Ingredients:
- ½ C. hot water
- 1 tsp. vanilla
- ¼ C. olive oil
- ½ C. almond milk
- 1 egg
- ½ tsp. salt
- ¾ tsp. baking soda
- ¾ tsp. baking powder
- ½ C. unsweetened cocoa powder
- 2 C. almond flour
- 1 C. brown sugar

Directions:
1. Preparing the Ingredients. Preheat your air fryer oven to 356 degrees.
2. Stir all dry ingredients together. Then stir in wet ingredients. Add hot water last.
3. The batter will be thin, no worries.
4. Air Frying. Pour cake batter into a pan that fits into the fryer. Cover with foil and poke holes into the foil.
5. Bake 35 minutes.
6. Discard foil and then bake another 10 minutes.
- **Nutrition Info:** CALORIES: 378; FAT:9G; PROTEIN:4G; SUGAR:5G

427.Caramelized Fruit Kebabs

Servings:4
Cooking Time: 4 Minutes
Ingredients:
- 2 peaches, peeled, pitted, and thickly sliced
- 3 plums, halved and pitted
- 3 nectarines, halved and pitted
- 1 tablespoon honey
- ½ teaspoon ground cinnamon
- ¼ teaspoon ground allspice
- Pinch cayenne pepper
- Special Equipment:
- 8 metal skewers

Directions:
1. Thread, alternating peaches, plums, and nectarines onto the metal skewers.
2. Thoroughly combine the honey, cinnamon, allspice, and cayenne in a small bowl. Brush generously the glaze over the fruit skewers.
3. Transfer the fruit skewers to the air fryer basket.
4. Put the air fryer basket on the baking pan and slide into Rack Position 2, select Air Fry, set temperature to 400ºF (205ºC), and set time to 4 minutes.

5. When cooking is complete, the fruit should be caramelized.
6. Remove the fruit skewers from the oven and let rest for 5 minutes before serving.

428.Mozzarella Sticks

Servings: 12 Sticks
Cooking Time: 15 Minutes
Ingredients:
- 6 (1-oz.mozzarella string cheese sticks
- ½ oz. pork rinds, finely ground
- 2 large eggs.
- ½ cup grated Parmesan cheese.
- 1 tsp. dried parsley.

Directions:
1. Place mozzarella sticks on a cutting board and cut in half. Freeze 45 minutes or until firm. If freezing overnight, remove frozen sticks after 1 hour and place into airtight zip-top storage bag and place back in freezer for future use.
2. Take a large bowl, mix Parmesan, ground pork rinds and parsley
3. Take a medium bowl, whisk eggs
4. Dip a frozen mozzarella stick into beaten eggs and then into Parmesan mixture to coat.
5. Repeat with remaining sticks. Place mozzarella sticks into the air fryer basket.
6. Adjust the temperature to 400 Degrees F and set the timer for 10 minutes or until golden. Serve warm.
- **Nutrition Info:** Calories: 236; Protein: 12g; Fiber: 0g; Fat: 18g; Carbs: 7g

429.Effortless Apple Pie

Servings: 4
Cooking Time: 30 Minutes
Ingredients:
- 4 apples, diced
- 2 oz butter, melted
- 2 oz sugar
- 1 oz brown sugar
- 2 tsp cinnamon
- 1 egg, beaten
- 3 large puff pastry sheets
- ¼ tsp salt

Directions:
1. Whisk white sugar, brown sugar, cinnamon, salt, and butter together. Place the apples in a greased baking pan and coat them with the sugar mixture. Place the baking dish in your and cook for 10 minutes at 350 F on Bake function.
2. Meanwhile, roll out the pastry on a floured flat surface, and cut each sheet into 6 equal pieces. Divide the apple filling between the pieces. Brush the edges of the pastry squares with the egg.

3. Fold them and seal the edges with a fork. Place on a lined baking sheet and cook in the fryer at 350 F for 8 minutes. Flip over, increase the temperature to 390 F, and cook for 2 more minutes.

430.Vanilla Rum Cookies With Walnuts

Servings: 6
Cooking Time: 15 Minutes
Ingredients:
- 1/2 cup almond flour
- 1/2 cup coconut flour
- 1/2 teaspoon baking powder
- 1/4 teaspoon fine sea salt
- 1 stick butter, unsalted and softened
- 1/2 cup swerve
- 1 egg
- 1/2 teaspoon vanilla
- 1 teaspoon butter rum flavoring
- 3 ounces walnuts, finely chopped

Directions:
1. Begin by preheating the Air Fryer to 360 degrees F.
2. In a mixing dish, thoroughly combine the flour with baking powder and salt.
3. Beat the butter and swerve with a hand mixer until pale and fluffy; add the whisked egg, vanilla, and butter rum flavoring; mix again to combine well. Now, stir in the dry ingredients.
4. Fold in the chopped walnuts and mix to combine. Divide the mixture into small balls; flatten each ball with a fork and transfer them to a foil-lined baking pan.
5. Bake in the preheated Air Fryer for 14 minutes. Work in a few batches and transfer to wire racks to cool completely.
- **Nutrition Info:** 314 Calories; 32g Fat; 7g Carbs; 2g Protein; 2g Sugars; 5g Fiber

431.Tomatoes Dip

Servings: 6
Cooking Time: 15 Minutes
Ingredients:
- 12 oz. cream cheese, soft
- 8 oz. mozzarella cheese; grated
- ¼ cup basil; chopped.
- ¼ cup parmesan; grated
- 4 garlic cloves; minced
- 1 pint grape tomatoes; halved
- 2 tbsp. thyme; chopped.
- ½ tbsp. oregano; chopped.
- 1 tsp. olive oil
- A pinch of salt and black pepper

Directions:
1. Put the tomatoes in your air fryer's basket and cook them at 400°F for 15 minutes.

2. In a blender, combine the fried tomatoes with the rest of the ingredients and pulse well
3. Transfer this to a ramekin, place it in the air fryer and cook at 400°F for 5 - 6 minutes more. Serve as a snack
- **Nutrition Info:** Calories: 184; Fat: 8g; Fiber: 3g; Carbs: 4g; Protein: 8g

432.Spicy Cauliflower Florets

Servings: 4
Cooking Time: 15 Minutes
Ingredients:
- 1 medium cauliflower head, cut into florets
- 1/2 tsp old bay seasoning
- 1/4 tsp paprika
- 1/4 tsp cayenne
- 1/4 tsp chili powder
- 1 tbsp garlic, minced
- 3 tbsp olive oil
- Pepper
- Salt

Directions:
1. Fit the oven with the rack in position 2.
2. In a bowl, toss cauliflower with remaining ingredients.
3. Add cauliflower florets in air fryer basket then place air fryer basket in baking pan.
4. Place a baking pan on the oven rack. Set to air fry at 400 F for 15 minutes.
5. Serve and enjoy.
- **Nutrition Info:** Calories 130 Fat 10.7 g Carbohydrates 8.6 g Sugar 3.5 g Protein 3 g Cholesterol 0 mg

433.Cream Caramel

Servings:x
Cooking Time:x
Ingredients:
- 3 tbsp. unsalted butter
- 4 tbsp. caramel
- 2 cups milk
- 2 cups custard powder
- 3 tbsp. powdered sugar

Directions:
1. Boil the milk and the sugar in a pan and add the custard powder and stir till you get a thick mixture.
2. Preheat the fryer to 300 Fahrenheit for five minutes. Place the dish in the basket and reduce the temperature to 250 Fahrenheit. Cook for ten minutes and set aside to cool.
3. Spread the caramel over the dish and serve warm.

434.Olive Tarts With Mushrooms

Servings:x
Cooking Time:x
Ingredients:

- ½ cup sliced black olives
- ½ cup sliced green olives
- ½ teaspoon dried thyme leaves
- 2 sheets frozen puff pastry, thawed
- 1 cup shredded Gouda cheese
- 1 onion, chopped
- 2 cloves garlic, minced
- ½ cup chopped mushrooms
- 1 tablespoon olive oil

Directions:
1. Preheat oven to 400ºF. In heavy skillet, sauté onion, garlic, and mushrooms in olive oil until tender. Remove from heat and add olives and thyme.
2. Gently roll puff pastry dough with rolling pin until ¼-inch thick. Using a 3-inch cookie cutter, cut 24 circles from pastry. Line muffin cups with dough.
3. Place a spoonful of filling in each pastry-lined cup. Bake at 400ºF for 10 to 12 minutes or until crust is golden brown and filling is set.
4. Remove from muffin cups and cool on wire rack. Flash freeze; when frozen solid, pack tarts into zipper-lock bags. Attach zipper-lock bag filled with shredded cheese; label and freeze.
5. To thaw and reheat: Thaw tarts in single layer overnight in refrigerator. Top each tart with cheese and bake at 400ºF for 5 to 6 minutes or until hot and cheese is melted.

435.Chocolate Chip Waffles

Servings:x
Cooking Time:x
Ingredients:
- Salt and Pepper to taste
- 3 tbsp. Butter
- 1 cup chocolate chips
- 3 cups cocoa powder
- 3 eggs
- 2 tsp. dried basil
- 2 tsp. dried parsley

Directions:
1. Preheat the air fryer to 250 Fahrenheit.
2. In a small bowl, mix the ingredients, except for the chocolate chips, together. Ensure that the mixture is smooth and well balanced. Take a waffle mold and grease it with butter. Add the batter to the mold and place it in the air fryer basket. Cook till both the sides have browned. Garnish with chips and serve.

436.Sausage And Onion Rolls

Servings:12
Cooking Time: 15 Minutes
Ingredients:
- 1 pound (454 g) bulk breakfast sausage

- ½ cup finely chopped onion
- ½ cup fresh bread crumbs
- ½ teaspoon dried mustard
- ½ teaspoon dried sage
- ¼ teaspoon cayenne pepper
- 1 large egg, beaten
- 1 garlic clove, minced
- 2 sheets (1 package) frozen puff pastry, thawed
- All-purpose flour, for dusting

Directions:
1. In a medium bowl, break up the sausage. Stir in the onion, bread crumbs, mustard, sage, cayenne pepper, egg and garlic. Divide the sausage mixture in half and tightly wrap each half in plastic wrap. Refrigerate for 5 to 10 minutes.
2. Lay the pastry sheets on a lightly floured work surface. Using a rolling pin, lightly roll out the pastry to smooth out the dough. Take out one of the sausage packages and form the sausage into a long roll. Remove the plastic wrap and place the sausage on top of the puff pastry about 1 inch from one of the long edges. Roll the pastry around the sausage and pinch the edges of the dough together to seal. Repeat with the other pastry sheet and sausage.
3. Slice the logs into lengths about 1½ inches long. Place the sausage rolls in the baking pan, cut-side down.
4. Slide the baking pan into Rack Position 2, select Roast, set temperature to 350ºF (180ºC) and set time to 15 minutes.
5. When cooking is complete, the rolls will be golden brown and sizzling. Remove from the oven and let cool for 5 minutes.

437.Garlicky Roasted Mushrooms

Servings:4
Cooking Time: 27 Minutes
Ingredients:
- 16 garlic cloves, peeled
- 2 teaspoons olive oil, divided
- 16 button mushrooms
- ½ teaspoon dried marjoram
- ⅛ teaspoon freshly ground black pepper
- 1 tablespoon white wine

Directions:
1. Place the garlic cloves in the baking pan and drizzle with 1 teaspoon of the olive oil. Toss to coat well.
2. Slide the baking pan into Rack Position 2, select Roast, set temperature to 350ºF (180ºC) and set time to 12 minutes.
3. When cooking is complete, remove from the oven. Stir in the mushrooms, marjoram and pepper. Drizzle with the remaining 1 teaspoon of the olive oil and the white wine.

Toss to coat well. Return the pan to the oven.
4. Select Roast, set temperature to 350ºF (180ºC) and set time to 15 minutes.
5. Once done, the mushrooms and garlic cloves will be softened. Remove from the oven.
6. Serve warm.

438.Mozzarella Pepperoni Pizza Bites

Servings:8
Cooking Time: 12 Minutes
Ingredients:
- 1 cup finely shredded Mozzarella cheese
- ½ cup chopped pepperoni
- ¼ cup Marinara sauce
- 1 (8-ounce / 227-g) can crescent roll dough
- All-purpose flour, for dusting

Directions:
1. In a small bowl, stir together the cheese, pepperoni and Marinara sauce.
2. Lay the dough on a lightly floured work surface. Separate it into 4 rectangles. Firmly pinch the perforations together and pat the dough pieces flat.
3. Divide the cheese mixture evenly between the rectangles and spread it out over the dough, leaving a ¼-inch border. Roll a rectangle up tightly, starting with the short end. Pinch the edge down to seal the roll. Repeat with the remaining rolls.
4. Slice the rolls into 4 or 5 even slices. Place the slices in the baking pan, leaving a few inches between each slice.
5. Slide the baking pan into Rack Position 2, select Roast, set temperature to 350ºF (180ºC) and set time to 12 minutes.
6. When cooking is complete, the rolls will be golden brown with crisp edges. Remove from the oven and serve hot.

439.Pistachio Pudding

Servings:x
Cooking Time:x
Ingredients:
- 3 tbsp. powdered sugar
- 3 tbsp. unsalted butter
- 2 cups milk
- 2 cups almond flour
- 2 tbsp. custard powder
- 2 cups finely chopped pistachio

Directions:
1. Boil the milk and the sugar in a pan and add the custard powder followed by the almond flour and stir till you get a thick mixture. Add the pistachio nuts to the mixture.
2. Preheat the fryer to 300 Fahrenheit for five minutes. Place the dish in the basket and

reduce the temperature to 250 Fahrenheit. Cook for ten minutes and set aside to cool.

440.Cheese Garlic Dip

Servings: 12
Cooking Time: 20 Minutes
Ingredients:
- 4 garlic cloves, minced
- 5 oz Asiago cheese, shredded
- 1 cup sour cream
- 1 cup mozzarella cheese, shredded
- 8 oz cream cheese, softened

Directions:
1. Fit the oven with the rack in position
2. Add all ingredients into the mixing bowl and mix until well combined.
3. Pour mixture into the baking dish.
4. Set to bake at 350 F for 25 minutes. After 5 minutes place the baking dish in the preheated oven.
5. Serve and enjoy.
- **Nutrition Info:** Calories 157 Fat 14.4 g Carbohydrates 1.7 g Sugar 0.1 g Protein 5.7 g Cholesterol 41 mg

441.Fried Pickles

Servings: 6
Cooking Time: 3 Minutes
Ingredients:
- Cold dill pickle slices, 36.
- Chopped fresh dill, 2 tbsps.
- Salt, 1 tsp.
- Divided cornstarch, 1 cup
- Ranch dressing
- Cayenne, ¼ tsp.
- Black pepper, 2 tsps.
- Almond meal, ½ cup
- Large egg, 1.
- Almond milk, ¾ cup
- Paprika, 2 tsps.
- Canola oil

Directions:
1. Whisk together cayenne, milk, and egg.
2. Spread half-cup cornstarch in a shallow dish.
3. Mix the remaining ½-cup cornstarch with almond meal, salt, pepper, dill, and paprika.
4. Dredge the pickle slices first through the cornstarch then dip them in an egg wash.
5. Coat them with almond meal mixture and shake off the excess.
6. Place them in the fryer basket and spray them with oil.
7. Return the basket to the fryer and air fry the pickles for 3 minutes at 3700 F working in batches as to not crowd the basket.
8. Serve warm.
- **Nutrition Info:** Calories: 138 Fat: 12.2 g Carbs: 5.8 g Protein: 4 g

442.Almond Pecan Cookies

Servings: 16
Cooking Time: 20 Minutes
Ingredients:
- 1/2 cup butter
- 1 tsp vanilla
- 2 tsp gelatin
- 2/3 cup Swerve
- 1 cup pecans
- 1/3 cup coconut flour
- 1 cup almond flour

Directions:
1. Fit the oven with the rack in position
2. Add butter, vanilla, gelatin, swerve, coconut flour, and almond flour into the food processor and process until crumbs form.
3. Add pecans and process until chopped.
4. Make cookies from prepared mixture and place onto a parchment-lined baking pan.
5. Set to bake at 350 F for 25 minutes. After 5 minutes place the baking pan in the preheated oven.
6. Serve and enjoy.
- **Nutrition Info:** Calories 101 Fat 10.2 g Carbohydrates 1.4 g Sugar 0.3 g Protein 1.8 g Cholesterol 15 mg

443.Delicious Cauliflower Hummus

Servings: 8
Cooking Time: 35 Minutes
Ingredients:
- 1 cauliflower head, cut into florets
- 3 tbsp olive oil
- 1/2 tsp ground cumin
- 2 tbsp fresh lemon juice
- 1/3 cup tahini
- 1 tsp garlic, chopped
- Pepper
- Salt

Directions:
1. Fit the oven with the rack in position
2. Spread cauliflower florets in baking pan.
3. Set to bake at 400 F for 40 minutes. After 5 minutes place the baking dish in the preheated oven.
4. Transfer roasted cauliflower into the food processor along with remaining ingredients and process until smooth.
5. Serve and enjoy.
- **Nutrition Info:** Calories 115 Fat 10.7 g Carbohydrates 4.2 g Sugar 0.9 g Protein 2.4 g Cholesterol 0 mg

444.Plum Cream(1)

Servings: 4
Cooking Time: 20 Minutes
Ingredients:
- 1-pound plums, pitted and chopped
- ¼ cup swerve

- 1 tablespoon lemon juice
- 1 and ½ cups heavy cream

Directions:
1. In a bowl, mix all the ingredients and whisk really well.
2. Divide this into 4 ramekins, put them in the air fryer and cook at 340 degrees F for 20 minutes.
3. Serve cold.
- **Nutrition Info:** calories 171, fat 4, fiber 2, carbs 4, protein 4

445.Sausage And Mushroom Empanadas

Servings:4
Cooking Time: 12 Minutes
Ingredients:
- ½ pound (227 g) Kielbasa smoked sausage, chopped
- 4 chopped canned mushrooms
- 2 tablespoons chopped onion
- ½ teaspoon ground cumin
- ¼ teaspoon paprika
- Salt and black pepper, to taste
- ½ package puff pastry dough, at room temperature
- 1 egg, beaten
- Cooking spray

Directions:
1. Combine the sausage, mushrooms, onion, cumin, paprika, salt, and pepper in a bowl and stir to mix well.
2. Make the empanadas: Place the puff pastry dough on a lightly floured surface. Cut circles into the dough with a glass. Place 1 tablespoon of the sausage mixture into the center of each pastry circle. Fold each in half and pinch the edges to seal. Using a fork, crimp the edges. Brush them with the beaten egg and mist with cooking spray.
3. Spritz the air fryer basket with cooking spray. Place the empanadas in the basket.
4. Put the air fryer basket on the baking pan and slide into Rack Position 2, select Air Fry, set temperature to 360ºF (182ºC), and set time to 12 minutes.
5. Flip the empanadas halfway through the cooking time.
6. When cooking is complete, the empanadas should be golden brown. Remove from the oven. Allow them to cool for 5 minutes and serve hot.

446.Delicious Banana Pastry With Berries

Servings:2
Cooking Time: 15 Minutes
Ingredients:
- 3 bananas, sliced
- 3 tbsp honey
- 2 puff pastry sheets, cut into thin strips
- Fresh berries to serve

Directions:
1. Preheat on AirFry function to 340 F. Place the banana slices into the cooking basket. Cover with the pastry strips and top with honey. Press Start and cook for 10-12 minutes on Bake function. Serve with fresh berries.

447.Pumpkin Bread

Servings: 10
Cooking Time: 40 Minutes
Ingredients:
- 1 1/3 cups all-purpose flour
- 1 cup sugar
- ¾ teaspoon baking soda
- 1 teaspoon pumpkin pie spice
- 1/3 teaspoon ground cinnamon
- ¼ teaspoon salt
- 2 eggs
- ½ cup pumpkin puree
- 1/3 cup vegetable oil
- ¼ cup water

Directions:
1. In a bowl, mix together the flour, sugar, baking soda, spices and salt
2. In another large bowl, add the eggs, pumpkin, oil and water and beat until well combined.
3. In a large mixing bowl or stand mixer.
4. Add the flour mixture and mix until just combined.
5. Place the mixture into a lightly greased loaf pan.
6. With a piece of foil, cover the pan loosely.
7. Press "Power Button" of Air Fry Oven and turn the dial to select the "Air Bake" mode.
8. Press the Time button and again turn the dial to set the cooking time to 40 minutes.
9. Now push the Temp button and rotate the dial to set the temperature at 325 degrees F.
10. Press "Start/Pause" button to start.
11. When the unit beeps to show that it is preheated, open the lid.
12. Arrange the pan in "Air Fry Basket" and insert in the oven.
13. After 25 minutes of cooking, remove the foil.
14. Place the pan onto a wire rack to cool for about 10 minutes.
15. Carefully, invert the bread onto wire rack to cool completely before slicing.
16. Cut the bread into desired-sized slices and serve.
- **Nutrition Info:** Calories 217 Total Fat 8.4 g Saturated Fat 1.4 g Cholesterol 33 mg Sodium 167 mg Total Carbs 34 g Fiber 0.9 g Sugar 20.5g Protein 3 g

448.Cranberry Pancakes

Servings:x
Cooking Time:x
Ingredients:
- 2 tsp. dried parsley
- Salt and Pepper to taste
- 3 tbsp. Butter
- 2 cups minced cranberry
- 1 ½ cups almond flour
- 3 eggs
- 2 tsp. dried basil

Directions:
1. Preheat the air fryer to 250 Fahrenheit.
2. In a small bowl, mix the ingredients together. Ensure that the mixture is smooth and well balanced.
3. Take a pancake mold and grease it with butter. Add the batter to the mold and place it in the air fryer basket. Cook till both the sides of the pancake have browned on both sides and serve with maple syrup.

449.Easy Pumpkin Pie

Servings: 8
Cooking Time: 35 Minutes
Ingredients:
- Egg yolks, 3.
- Large egg, 1.
- Ground ginger, ½ tsp.
- Fine salt, ½ tsp.
- Chinese 5-spice powder, 1/8 tsp.
- Unbaked pie crust, 19-inch.
- Freshly grated nutmeg, ¼ tsp.
- Sweetened condensed milk, 14 oz.
- Pumpkin puree, 15 oz.
- Ground cinnamon, 1 tsp.

Directions:
1. Lightly grease a baking pan of air fryer with cooking spray. Press pie crust on bottom of pan, stretching all the way up to the sides of the pan. Pierce all over with a fork.
2. In blender, blend well egg, egg yolks, and pumpkin puree. Add Chinese 5-spice powder, nutmeg, salt, ginger, cinnamon, and condensed milk. Pour on top of pie crust.
3. Cover pan with foil.
4. For 15 minutes, cook on preheated 390 °F air fryer.
5. Cook for 20 more minutes at 330 °F without the foil until middle is set.
6. Allow to cool in air fryer completely.
7. Serve and enjoy.
- **Nutrition Info:** Calories: 326 Carbs: 41.9g Fat: 14.2g Protein: 7.6g

450.Chocolate Cheesecake

Servings:6
Cooking Time: 18 Minutes
Ingredients:
- Crust:
- ½ cup butter, melted
- ½ cup coconut flour
- 2 tablespoons stevia
- Cooking spray
- Topping:
- 4 ounces (113 g) unsweetened baker's chocolate
- 1 cup mascarpone cheese, at room temperature
- 1 teaspoon vanilla extract
- 2 drops peppermint extract

Directions:
1. Lightly coat the baking pan with cooking spray.
2. In a mixing bowl, whisk together the butter, flour, and stevia until well combined. Transfer the mixture to the prepared baking pan.
3. Slide the baking pan into Rack Position 1, select Convection Bake, set temperature to 350ºF (180ºC), and set time to 18 minutes.
4. When done, a toothpick inserted in the center should come out clean.
5. Remove the crust from the oven to a wire rack to cool.
6. Once cooled completely, place it in the freezer for 20 minutes.
7. When ready, combine all the ingredients for the topping in a small bowl and stir to incorporate.
8. Spread this topping over the crust and let it sit for another 15 minutes in the freezer.
9. Serve chilled.

451.Beefy Mini Pies

Servings:x
Cooking Time:x
Ingredients:
- 1 cup shredded Colby cheese
- 2 eggs
- ½ cup half-and-half
- ½ teaspoon dried dill weed
- 1 (10-ounce) package refrigerated flaky dinner rolls
- ½ pound ground beef
- 1 small onion, chopped
- 2 cloves garlic, minced

Directions:
1. Preheat oven to 350ºF. Remove rolls from package and divide each roll into 3 rounds. Place each round into a 3-inch muffin cup; press firmly onto bottom and up sides.
2. In a heavy skillet, cook ground beef with onion and garlic until beef is done. Drain well. Place 1 tablespoon beef mixture into each dough-lined muffin cup. Sprinkle cheese over beef mixture. In a small bowl, beat together eggs, half-and-half, and dill

weed. Spoon this mixture over beef in muffin cups, making sure not to overfill cups.

3. Bake at 350ºF for 10 to 13 minutes or until filling is puffed and set. Flash freeze in single layer on baking sheet. When frozen solid, wrap, label, and freeze.
4. To thaw and reheat: Thaw pies in single layer in refrigerator overnight. Bake at 350ºF for 7 to 9 minutes or until hot.

452.Cajun Sweet Potato Tots

Servings: 24
Cooking Time: 8 Minutes
Ingredients:
- 1/2 tsp Cajun seasoning
- 2 sweet potatoes, peeled
- Salt

Directions:
1. Fit the oven with the rack in position 2.
2. Add water in a large pot and bring to boil.
3. Add sweet potatoes to the pot and boil for 15 minutes. Drain well.
4. Grated boil sweet potatoes into a large bowl using a grated.
5. Add Cajun seasoning and salt in grated sweet potatoes and mix until well combined.
6. Make a small tot of sweet potato mixture and place in the air fryer basket then place an air fryer basket in the baking pan.
7. Place a baking pan on the oven rack. Set to air fry at 400 F for 8 minutes.
8. Serve and enjoy.
- **Nutrition Info:** Calories 10 Fat 0 g Carbohydrates 2.3 g Sugar 0 g Protein 0.1 g Cholesterol 0 mg

453.Easy Bacon Bites

Servings: 4
Cooking Time: 10 Minutes
Ingredients:
- 4 bacon strips, cut into small pieces
- 1/4 cup hot sauce
- 1/2 cup pork rinds, crushed

Directions:
1. Fit the oven with the rack in position 2.
2. Add bacon pieces in a bowl.
3. Add hot sauce and toss well.
4. Add crushed pork rinds and toss until bacon pieces are well coated.
5. Transfer bacon pieces in the air fryer basket then place an air fryer basket in the baking pan.
6. Place a baking pan on the oven rack. Set to air fry at 350 F for 10 minutes.
7. Serve and enjoy.
- **Nutrition Info:** Calories 123 Fat 10.4 g Carbohydrates 0.3 g Sugar 0.2 g Protein 6.5 g Cholesterol 5 mg

454.Classic Pound Cake

Servings:8
Cooking Time: 30 Minutes
Ingredients:
- 1 stick butter, at room temperature
- 1 cup Swerve
- 4 eggs
- 1½ cups coconut flour
- ½ cup buttermilk
- ½ teaspoon baking soda
- ½ teaspoon baking powder
- ¼ teaspoon salt
- 1 teaspoon vanilla essence
- A pinch of ground star anise
- A pinch of freshly grated nutmeg
- Cooking spray

Directions:
1. Spray the baking pan with cooking spray.
2. With an electric mixer or hand mixer, beat the butter and Swerve until creamy. One at a time, mix in the eggs and whisk until fluffy. Add the remaining ingredients and stir to combine.
3. Transfer the batter to the prepared baking pan.
4. Slide the baking pan into Rack Position 1, select Convection Bake, set temperature to 320ºF (160ºC), and set time to 30 minutes.
5. When cooking is complete, the center of the cake should be springy.
6. Allow the cake to cool in the pan for 10 minutes before removing and serving.

455.Apple Hand Pies

Servings: 6
Cooking Time: 8 Minutes
Ingredients:
- 15-ounces no-sugar-added apple pie filling
- 1 store-bought crust

Directions:
1. Preparing the Ingredients. Lay out pie crust and slice into equal-sized squares.
2. Place 2 tbsp. filling into each square and seal crust with a fork.
3. Air Frying. Place into the air fryer oven. Cook 8 minutes at 390 degrees until golden in color.
- **Nutrition Info:** CALORIES: 278; FAT:10G; PROTEIN:5G; SUGAR:4G

456.Cheesy Crab Toasts

Servings: 15 To 18 Toasts
Cooking Time: 5 Minutes
Ingredients:
- 1 (6-ounce / 170-g) can flaked crab meat, well drained
- 3 tablespoons light mayonnaise
- ¼ cup shredded Parmesan cheese
- ¼ cup shredded Cheddar cheese

- 1 teaspoon Worcestershire sauce
- ½ teaspoon lemon juice
- 1 loaf artisan bread, French bread, or baguette, cut into ⅜-inch-thick slices

Directions:
1. In a large bowl, stir together all the ingredients except the bread slices.
2. On a clean work surface, lay the bread slices. Spread ½ tablespoon of crab mixture onto each slice of bread.
3. Arrange the bread slices in the baking pan in a single layer.
4. Slide the baking pan into Rack Position 1, select Convection Bake, set temperature to 360ºF (182ºC), and set time to 5 minutes.
5. When cooking is complete, the tops should be lightly browned. Remove from the oven and serve warm.

OTHER FAVORITE RECIPES

457.Enchilada Sauce

Servings: 2 Cups
Cooking Time: 0 Minutes
Ingredients:
- 3 large ancho chiles, stems and seeds removed, torn into pieces
- 1½ cups very hot water
- 2 garlic cloves, peeled and lightly smashed
- 2 tablespoons wine vinegar
- 1½ teaspoons sugar
- ½ teaspoon dried oregano
- ½ teaspoon ground cumin
- 2 teaspoons kosher salt or 1 teaspoon fine salt

Directions:
1. Mix together the chile pieces and hot water in a bowl and let stand for 10 to 15 minutes.
2. Pour the chiles and water into a blender jar. Fold in the garlic, vinegar, sugar, oregano, cumin, and salt and blend until smooth.
3. Use immediately.

458.Herbed Cheddar Frittata

Servings:4
Cooking Time: 20 Minutes
Ingredients:
- ½ cup shredded Cheddar cheese
- ½ cup half-and-half
- 4 large eggs
- 2 tablespoons chopped scallion greens
- 2 tablespoons chopped fresh parsley
- ½ teaspoon kosher salt
- ½ teaspoon ground black pepper
- Cooking spray

Directions:
1. Spritz the baking pan with cooking spray.
2. Whisk together all the ingredients in a large bowl, then pour the mixture into the prepared baking pan.
3. Slide the baking pan into Rack Position 1, select Convection Bake, set temperature to 300ºF (150ºC) and set time to 20 minutes.
4. Stir the mixture halfway through.
5. When cooking is complete, the eggs should be set.
6. Serve immediately.

459.Milky Pecan Tart

Servings:8
Cooking Time: 26 Minutes
Ingredients:
- Tart Crust:
- ¼ cup firmly packed brown sugar
- $^{1}/_{3}$ cup butter, softened
- 1 cup all-purpose flour
- ¼ teaspoon kosher salt
- Filling:
- ¼ cup whole milk
- 4 tablespoons butter, diced
- ½ cup packed brown sugar
- ¼ cup pure maple syrup
- 1½ cups finely chopped pecans
- ¼ teaspoon pure vanilla extract
- ¼ teaspoon sea salt

Directions:
1. Line the baking pan with aluminum foil, then spritz the pan with cooking spray.
2. Stir the brown sugar and butter in a bowl with a hand mixer until puffed, then add the flour and salt and stir until crumbled.
3. Pour the mixture in the prepared baking pan and tilt the pan to coat the bottom evenly.
4. Slide the baking pan into Rack Position 1, select Convection Bake, set temperature to 350ºF (180ºC) and set time to 13 minutes.
5. When done, the crust will be golden brown.
6. Meanwhile, pour the milk, butter, sugar, and maple syrup in a saucepan. Stir to mix well. Bring to a simmer, then cook for 1 more minute. Stir constantly.
7. Turn off the heat and mix the pecans and vanilla into the filling mixture.
8. Pour the filling mixture over the golden crust and spread with a spatula to coat the crust evenly.
9. Select Bake and set time to 12 minutes. When cooked, the filling mixture should be set and frothy.
10. Remove the baking pan from the oven and sprinkle with salt. Allow to sit for 10 minutes or until cooled.
11. Transfer the pan to the refrigerator to chill for at least 2 hours, then remove the aluminum foil and slice to serve.

460.Parmesan Cauliflower Fritters

Servings:6
Cooking Time: 8 Minutes
Ingredients:
- 2 cups cooked cauliflower
- 1 cup panko bread crumbs
- 1 large egg, beaten
- ½ cup grated Parmesan cheese
- 1 tablespoon chopped fresh chives Spritz the air fryer basket with cooking spray
- Cooking spray.

Directions:
1. Put the cauliflower, panko bread crumbs, egg, Parmesan, and chives in a food processor, then pulse to lightly mash and combine the mixture until chunky and thick.

2. Shape the mixture into 6 flat patties, then arrange them in the basket and spritz with cooking spray.
3. Put the air fryer basket on the baking pan and slide into Rack Position 2, select Air Fry, set temperature to 390ºF (199ºC) and set time to 8 minutes.
4. Flip the patties halfway through the cooking time.
5. When done, the patties should be crispy and golden brown. Remove from the oven and serve immediately.

461.Easy Corn And Bell Pepper Casserole

Servings:4
Cooking Time: 20 Minutes
Ingredients:
- 1 cup corn kernels
- ¼ cup bell pepper, finely chopped
- ½ cup low-fat milk
- 1 large egg, beaten
- ½ cup yellow cornmeal
- ½ cup all-purpose flour
- ½ teaspoon baking powder
- 2 tablespoons melted unsalted butter
- 1 tablespoon granulated sugar
- Pinch of cayenne pepper
- ¼ teaspoon kosher salt
- Cooking spray

Directions:
1. Spritz the baking pan with cooking spray.
2. Combine all the ingredients in a large bowl. Stir to mix well. Pour the mixture into the baking pan.
3. Slide the baking pan into Rack Position 1, select Convection Bake, set temperature to 330ºF (166ºC) and set time to 20 minutes.
4. When cooking is complete, the casserole should be lightly browned and set.
5. Remove from the oven and serve immediately.

462.Shrimp Spinach Frittata

Servings:4
Cooking Time: 14 Minutes
Ingredients:
- 4 whole eggs
- 1 teaspoon dried basil
- ½ cup shrimp, cooked and chopped
- ½ cup baby spinach
- ½ cup rice, cooked
- ½ cup Monterey Jack cheese, grated
- Salt, to taste
- Cooking spray

Directions:
1. Spritz the baking pan with cooking spray.
2. Whisk the eggs with basil and salt in a large bowl until bubbly, then mix in the shrimp, spinach, rice, and cheese.

3. Pour the mixture into the baking pan.
4. Slide the baking pan into Rack Position 1, select Convection Bake, set temperature to 360ºF (182ºC) and set time to 14 minutes.
5. Stir the mixture halfway through.
6. When cooking is complete, the eggs should be set and the frittata should be golden brown.
7. Slice to serve.

463.Sausage And Colorful Peppers Casserole

Servings:6
Cooking Time: 25 Minutes
Ingredients:
- 1 pound (454 g) minced breakfast sausage
- 1 yellow pepper, diced
- 1 red pepper, diced
- 1 green pepper, diced
- 1 sweet onion, diced
- 2 cups Cheddar cheese, shredded
- 6 eggs
- Salt and freshly ground black pepper, to taste
- Fresh parsley, for garnish

Directions:
1. Cook the sausage in a nonstick skillet over medium heat for 10 minutes or until well browned. Stir constantly.
2. When the cooking is finished, transfer the cooked sausage to the baking pan and add the peppers and onion. Scatter with Cheddar cheese.
3. Whisk the eggs with salt and ground black pepper in a large bowl, then pour the mixture into the baking pan.
4. Slide the baking pan into Rack Position 1, select Convection Bake, set temperature to 360ºF (182ºC) and set time to 15 minutes.
5. When cooking is complete, the egg should be set and the edges of the casserole should be lightly browned.
6. Remove from the oven and top with fresh parsley before serving.

464.Bartlett Pears With Lemony Ricotta

Servings:4
Cooking Time: 8 Minutes
Ingredients:
- 2 large Bartlett pears, peeled, cut in half, cored
- 3 tablespoons melted butter
- ½ teaspoon ground ginger
- ¼ teaspoon ground cardamom
- 3 tablespoons brown sugar
- ½ cup whole-milk ricotta cheese
- 1 teaspoon pure lemon extract
- 1 teaspoon pure almond extract

- 1 tablespoon honey, plus additional for drizzling

Directions:

1. Toss the pears with butter, ginger, cardamom, and sugar in a large bowl. Toss to coat well. Arrange the pears in the baking pan, cut side down.
2. Put the air fryer basket on the baking pan and slide into Rack Position 2, select Air Fry, set temperature to 375ºF (190ºC) and set time to 8 minutes.
3. After 5 minutes, remove the pan and flip the pears. Return to the oven and continue cooking.
4. When cooking is complete, the pears should be soft and browned. Remove from the oven.
5. In the meantime, combine the remaining ingredients in a separate bowl. Whip for 1 minute with a hand mixer until the mixture is puffed.
6. Divide the mixture into four bowls, then put the pears over the mixture and drizzle with more honey to serve.

465.Ritzy Pimento And Almond Turkey Casserole

Servings:4
Cooking Time: 32 Minutes
Ingredients:

- 1 pound (454 g) turkey breasts
- 1 tablespoon olive oil
- 2 boiled eggs, chopped
- 2 tablespoons chopped pimentos
- ¼ cup slivered almonds, chopped
- ¼ cup mayonnaise
- ½ cup diced celery
- 2 tablespoons chopped green onion
- ¼ cup cream of chicken soup
- ¼ cup bread crumbs
- Salt and ground black pepper, to taste

Directions:

1. Put the turkey breasts in a large bowl. Sprinkle with salt and ground black pepper and drizzle with olive oil. Toss to coat well.
2. Transfer the turkey to the air fryer basket.
3. Put the air fryer basket on the baking pan and slide into Rack Position 2, select Air Fry, set temperature to 390ºF (199ºC) and set time to 12 minutes.
4. Flip the turkey halfway through.
5. When cooking is complete, the turkey should be well browned.
6. Remove the turkey breasts from the oven and cut into cubes, then combine the chicken cubes with eggs, pimentos, almonds, mayo, celery, green onions, and chicken soup in a large bowl. Stir to mix.
7. Pour the mixture into the baking pan, then spread with bread crumbs.

8. Slide the baking pan into Rack Position 1, select Convection Bake, set time to 20 minutes.
9. When cooking is complete, the eggs should be set.
10. Remove from the oven and serve immediately.

466.Ritzy Chicken And Vegetable Casserole

Servings:4
Cooking Time: 15 Minutes
Ingredients:

- 4 boneless and skinless chicken breasts, cut into cubes
- 2 carrots, sliced
- 1 yellow bell pepper, cut into strips
- 1 red bell pepper, cut into strips
- 15 ounces (425 g) broccoli florets
- 1 cup snow peas
- 1 scallion, sliced
- Cooking spray
- Sauce:
- 1 teaspoon Sriracha
- 3 tablespoons soy sauce
- 2 tablespoons oyster sauce
- 1 tablespoon rice wine vinegar
- 1 teaspoon cornstarch
- 1 tablespoon grated ginger
- 2 garlic cloves, minced
- 1 teaspoon sesame oil
- 1 tablespoon brown sugar

Directions:

1. Spritz the baking pan with cooking spray.
2. Combine the chicken, carrot, and bell peppers in a large bowl. Stir to mix well.
3. Combine the ingredients for the sauce in a separate bowl. Stir to mix well.
4. Pour the chicken mixture into the baking pan, then pour the sauce over. Stir to coat well.
5. Slide the baking pan into Rack Position 1, select Convection Bake, set temperature to 370ºF (188ºC) and set time to 13 minutes.
6. Add the broccoli and snow peas to the pan halfway through.
7. When cooking is complete, the vegetables should be tender.
8. Remove from the oven and sprinkle with sliced scallion before serving.

467.Cheesy Green Bean Casserole

Servings:4
Cooking Time: 6 Minutes
Ingredients:

- 1 tablespoon melted butter
- 1 cup green beans
- 6 ounces (170 g) Cheddar cheese, shredded

- 7 ounces (198 g) Parmesan cheese, shredded
- ¼ cup heavy cream
- Sea salt, to taste

Directions:
1. Grease the baking pan with the melted butter.
2. Add the green beans, Cheddar, salt, and black pepper to the prepared baking pan. Stir to mix well, then spread the Parmesan and cream on top.
3. Slide the baking pan into Rack Position 1, select Convection Bake, set temperature to 400ºF (205ºC) and set time to 6 minutes.
4. When cooking is complete, the beans should be tender and the cheese should be melted.
5. Serve immediately.

468.Chicken Divan

Servings:4
Cooking Time: 24 Minutes
Ingredients:
- 4 chicken breasts
- Salt and ground black pepper, to taste
- 1 head broccoli, cut into florets
- ½ cup cream of mushroom soup
- 1 cup shredded Cheddar cheese
- ½ cup croutons
- Cooking spray

Directions:
1. Spritz the air fryer basket with cooking spray.
2. Put the chicken breasts in the basket and sprinkle with salt and ground black pepper.
3. Put the air fryer basket on the baking pan and slide into Rack Position 2, select Air Fry, set temperature to 390ºF (199ºC) and set time to 14 minutes.
4. Flip the breasts halfway through the cooking time.
5. When cooking is complete, the breasts should be well browned and tender.
6. Remove the breasts from the oven and allow to cool for a few minutes on a plate, then cut the breasts into bite-size pieces.
7. Combine the chicken, broccoli, mushroom soup, and Cheddar cheese in a large bowl. Stir to mix well.
8. Spritz the baking pan with cooking spray. Pour the chicken mixture into the pan. Spread the croutons over the mixture.
9. Slide the baking pan into Rack Position 1, select Convection Bake, set time to 10 minutes.
10. When cooking is complete, the croutons should be lightly browned and the mixture should be set.
11. Remove from the oven and serve immediately.

469.Chocolate Buttermilk Cake

Servings:8
Cooking Time: 20 Minutes
Ingredients:
- 1 cup all-purpose flour
- $^2/_3$ cup granulated white sugar
- ¼ cup unsweetened cocoa powder
- ¾ teaspoon baking soda
- ¼ teaspoon salt
- $^2/_3$ cup buttermilk
- 2 tablespoons plus 2 teaspoons vegetable oil
- 1 teaspoon vanilla extract
- Cooking spray

Directions:
1. Spritz the baking pan with cooking spray.
2. Combine the flour, cocoa powder, baking soda, sugar, and salt in a large bowl. Stir to mix well.
3. Mix in the buttermilk, vanilla, and vegetable oil. Keep stirring until it forms a grainy and thick dough.
4. Scrape the chocolate batter from the bowl and transfer to the pan, level the batter in an even layer with a spatula.
5. Slide the baking pan into Rack Position 1, select Convection Bake, set temperature to 325ºF (163ºC) and set time to 20 minutes.
6. After 15 minutes, remove the pan from the oven. Check the doneness. Return the pan to the oven and continue cooking.
7. When done, a toothpick inserted in the center should come out clean.
8. Invert the cake on a cooling rack and allow to cool for 15 minutes before slicing to serve.

470.Smoked Trout And Crème Fraiche Frittata

Servings:4
Cooking Time: 17 Minutes
Ingredients:
- 2 tablespoons olive oil
- 1 onion, sliced
- 1 egg, beaten
- ½ tablespoon horseradish sauce
- 6 tablespoons crème fraiche
- 1 cup diced smoked trout
- 2 tablespoons chopped fresh dill
- Cooking spray

Directions:
1. Spritz the baking pan with cooking spray.
2. Heat the olive oil in a nonstick skillet over medium heat until shimmering.
3. Add the onion and sauté for 3 minutes or until translucent.
4. Combine the egg, horseradish sauce, and crème fraiche in a large bowl. Stir to mix

well, then mix in the sautéed onion, smoked trout, and dill.

5. Pour the mixture in the prepared baking pan.
6. Slide the baking pan into Rack Position 1, select Convection Bake, set temperature to 350ºF (180ºC) and set time to 14 minutes.
7. Stir the mixture halfway through.
8. When cooking is complete, the egg should be set and the edges should be lightly browned.
9. Serve immediately.

471. Crunchy Green Tomatoes Slices

Servings: 12 Slices
Cooking Time: 8 Minutes
Ingredients:
- ½ cup all-purpose flour
- 1 egg
- ½ cup buttermilk
- 1 cup cornmeal
- 1 cup panko
- 2 green tomatoes, cut into ¼-inch-thick slices, patted dry
- ½ teaspoon salt
- ½ teaspoon ground black pepper
- Cooking spray

Directions:
1. Spritz a baking sheet with cooking spray.
2. Pour the flour in a bowl. Whisk the egg and buttermilk in a second bowl. Combine the cornmeal and panko in a third bowl.
3. Dredge the tomato slices in the bowl of flour first, then into the egg mixture, and then dunk the slices into the cornmeal mixture. Shake the excess off.
4. Transfer the well-coated tomato slices in the baking sheet and sprinkle with salt and ground black pepper. Spritz the tomato slices with cooking spray.
5. Put the air fryer basket on the baking pan and slide into Rack Position 2, select Air Fry, set temperature to 400ºF (205ºC) and set time to 8 minutes.
6. Flip the slices halfway through the cooking time.
7. When cooking is complete, the tomato slices should be crispy and lightly browned. Remove the baking sheet from the oven.
8. Serve immediately.

472. Sumptuous Vegetable Frittata

Servings: 2
Cooking Time: 20 Minutes
Ingredients:
- 4 eggs
- ¹/₃ cup milk
- 2 teaspoons olive oil
- 1 large zucchini, sliced
- 2 asparagus, sliced thinly
- ¹/₃ cup sliced mushrooms
- 1 cup baby spinach
- 1 small red onion, sliced
- ¹/₃ cup crumbled feta cheese
- ¹/₃ cup grated Cheddar cheese
- ¼ cup chopped chives
- Salt and ground black pepper, to taste

Directions:
1. Line the baking pan with parchment paper.
2. Whisk together the eggs, milk, salt, and ground black pepper in a large bowl. Set aside.
3. Heat the olive oil in a nonstick skillet over medium heat until shimmering.
4. Add the zucchini, asparagus, mushrooms, spinach, and onion to the skillet and sauté for 5 minutes or until tender.
5. Pour the sautéed vegetables into the prepared baking pan, then spread the egg mixture over and scatter with cheeses.
6. Slide the baking pan into Rack Position 1, select Convection Bake, set temperature to 380ºF (193ºC) and set time to 15 minutes.
7. Stir the mixture halfway through.
8. When cooking is complete, the egg should be set and the edges should be lightly browned.
9. Remove the frittata from the oven and sprinkle with chives before serving.

473. Classic Marinara Sauce

Servings: About 3 Cups
Cooking Time: 30 Minutes
Ingredients:
- ¼ cup extra-virgin olive oil
- 3 garlic cloves, minced
- 1 small onion, chopped (about ½ cup)
- 2 tablespoons minced or puréed sun-dried tomatoes (optional)
- 1 (28-ounce / 794-g) can crushed tomatoes
- ½ teaspoon dried basil
- ½ teaspoon dried oregano
- ¼ teaspoon red pepper flakes

Directions:
1. 1 teaspoon kosher salt or ½ teaspoon fine salt, plus more as needed
2. Heat the oil in a medium saucepan over medium heat.
3. Add the garlic and onion and sauté for 2 to 3 minutes, or until the onion is softened. Add the sun-dried tomatoes (if desired) and cook for 1 minute until fragrant. Stir in the crushed tomatoes, scraping any brown bits from the bottom of the pot. Fold in the basil, oregano, red pepper flakes, and salt. Stir well.
4. Bring to a simmer. Cook covered for about 30 minutes, stirring occasionally.

5. Turn off the heat and allow the sauce to cool for about 10 minutes.
6. Taste and adjust the seasoning, adding more salt if needed.
7. Use immediately.

474.Asian Dipping Sauce

Servings: About 1 Cup
Cooking Time: 0 Minutes
Ingredients:
- ¼ cup rice vinegar
- ¼ cup hoisin sauce
- ¼ cup low-sodium chicken or vegetable stock
- 3 tablespoons soy sauce
- 1 tablespoon minced or grated ginger
- 1 tablespoon minced or pressed garlic
- 1 teaspoon chili-garlic sauce or sriracha (or more to taste)

Directions:
1. Stir together all the ingredients in a small bowl, or place in a jar with a tight-fitting lid and shake until well mixed.
2. Use immediately.

475.Roasted Carrot Chips

Servings: 3 Cups
Cooking Time: 15 Minutes
Ingredients:
- 3 large carrots, peeled and sliced into long and thick chips diagonally
- 1 tablespoon granulated garlic
- 1 teaspoon salt
- ¼ teaspoon ground black pepper
- 1 tablespoon olive oil
- 1 tablespoon finely chopped fresh parsley

Directions:
1. Toss the carrots with garlic, salt, ground black pepper, and olive oil in a large bowl to coat well. Place the carrots in the air fryer basket.
2. Put the air fryer basket on the baking pan and slide into Rack Position 2, select Roast, set temperature to 360ºF (182ºC) and set time to 15 minutes.
3. Stir the carrots halfway through the cooking time.
4. When cooking is complete, the carrot chips should be soft. Remove from the oven. Serve the carrot chips with parsley on top.

476.Pão De Queijo

Servings: 12 Balls
Cooking Time: 12 Minutes
Ingredients:
- 2 tablespoons butter, plus more for greasing
- ½ cup milk
- 1½ cups tapioca flour
- ½ teaspoon salt
- 1 large egg
- $^2/_3$ cup finely grated aged Asiago cheese

Directions:
1. Put the butter in a saucepan and pour in the milk, heat over medium heat until the liquid boils. Keep stirring.
2. Turn off the heat and mix in the tapioca flour and salt to form a soft dough. Transfer the dough in a large bowl, then wrap the bowl in plastic and let sit for 15 minutes.
3. Break the egg in the bowl of dough and whisk with a hand mixer for 2 minutes or until a sanity dough forms. Fold the cheese in the dough. Cover the bowl in plastic again and let sit for 10 more minutes.
4. Grease the baking pan with butter.
5. Scoop 2 tablespoons of the dough into the baking pan. Repeat with the remaining dough to make dough 12 balls. Keep a little distance between each two balls.
6. Slide the baking pan into Rack Position 1, select Convection Bake, set temperature to 375ºF (190ºC) and set time to 12 minutes.
7. Flip the balls halfway through the cooking time.
8. When cooking is complete, the balls should be golden brown and fluffy.
9. Remove the balls from the oven and allow to cool for 5 minutes before serving.

477.Crunchy And Beery Onion Rings

Servings:2 To 4
Cooking Time: 16 Minutes
Ingredients:
- $^2/_3$ cup all-purpose flour
- 1 teaspoon paprika
- ½ teaspoon baking soda
- 1 teaspoon salt
- ½ teaspoon freshly ground black pepper
- 1 egg, beaten
- ¾ cup beer
- 1½ cups bread crumbs
- 1 tablespoons olive oil
- 1 large Vidalia onion, peeled and sliced into ½-inch rings
- Cooking spray

Directions:
1. Spritz the air fryer basket with cooking spray.
2. Combine the flour, paprika, baking soda, salt, and ground black pepper in a bowl. Stir to mix well.
3. Combine the egg and beer in a separate bowl. Stir to mix well.
4. Make a well in the center of the flour mixture, then pour the egg mixture in the well. Stir to mix everything well.

5. Pour the bread crumbs and olive oil in a shallow plate. Stir to mix well.
6. Dredge the onion rings gently into the flour and egg mixture, then shake the excess off and put into the plate of bread crumbs. Flip to coat the both sides well. Arrange the onion rings in the basket.
7. Put the air fryer basket on the baking pan and slide into Rack Position 2, select Air Fry, set temperature to 360ºF (182ºC) and set time to 16 minutes.
8. Flip the rings and put the bottom rings to the top halfway through.
9. When cooked, the rings will be golden brown and crunchy. Remove from the oven and serve immediately.

478.Sweet Air Fried Pecans

Servings: 4 Cups
Cooking Time: 10 Minutes
Ingredients:
- 2 egg whites
- 1 tablespoon cumin
- 2 teaspoons smoked paprika
- ½ cup brown sugar
- 2 teaspoons kosher salt
- 1 pound (454 g) pecan halves
- Cooking spray

Directions:
1. Spritz the air fryer basket with cooking spray.
2. Combine the egg whites, cumin, paprika, sugar, and salt in a large bowl. Stir to mix well. Add the pecans to the bowl and toss to coat well.
3. Transfer the pecans to the basket.
4. Put the air fryer basket on the baking pan and slide into Rack Position 2, select Air Fry, set temperature to 300ºF (150ºC) and set time to 10 minutes.
5. Stir the pecans at least two times during the cooking.
6. When cooking is complete, the pecans should be lightly caramelized. Remove from the oven and serve immediately.

479.South Carolina Shrimp And Corn Bake

Servings:2
Cooking Time: 18 Minutes
Ingredients:
- 1 ear corn, husk and silk removed, cut into 2-inch rounds
- 8 ounces (227 g) red potatoes, unpeeled, cut into 1-inch pieces
- 2 teaspoons Old Bay Seasoning, divided
- 2 teaspoons vegetable oil, divided
- ¼ teaspoon ground black pepper
- 8 ounces (227 g) large shrimps (about 12 shrimps), deveined

- 6 ounces (170 g) andouille or chorizo sausage, cut into 1-inch pieces
- 2 garlic cloves, minced
- 1 tablespoon chopped fresh parsley

Directions:
1. Put the corn rounds and potatoes in a large bowl. Sprinkle with 1 teaspoon of Old Bay seasoning and drizzle with vegetable oil. Toss to coat well.
2. Transfer the corn rounds and potatoes into the baking pan.
3. Slide the baking pan into Rack Position 1, select Convection Bake, set temperature to 400ºF (205ºC) and set time to 18 minutes.
4. After 6 minutes, remove from the oven. Stir the corn rounds and potatoes. Return the pan to the oven and continue cooking.
5. Meanwhile, cut slits into the shrimps but be careful not to cut them through. Combine the shrimps, sausage, remaining Old Bay seasoning, and remaining vegetable oil in the large bowl. Toss to coat well.
6. After 6 minutes, remove the pan from the oven. Add the shrimps and sausage to the pan. Return the pan to the oven and continue cooking for 6 minutes. Stir the shrimp mixture halfway through the cooking time.
7. When done, the shrimps should be opaque. Transfer the dish to a plate and spread with parsley before serving.

480.Southwest Corn And Bell Pepper Roast

Servings:4
Cooking Time: 10 Minutes
Ingredients:
- Corn:
- 1½ cups thawed frozen corn kernels
- 1 cup mixed diced bell peppers
- 1 jalapeño, diced
- 1 cup diced yellow onion
- ½ teaspoon ancho chile powder
- 1 tablespoon fresh lemon juice
- 1 teaspoon ground cumin
- ½ teaspoon kosher salt
- Cooking spray
- For Serving:
- ¼ cup feta cheese
- ¼ cup chopped fresh cilantro
- 1 tablespoon fresh lemon juice

Directions:
1. Spritz the air fryer basket with cooking spray.
2. Combine the ingredients for the corn in a large bowl. Stir to mix well.
3. Pour the mixture into the basket.
4. Put the air fryer basket on the baking pan and slide into Rack Position 2, select Air Fry,

set temperature to 375ºF (190ºC) and set time to 10 minutes.

5. Stir the mixture halfway through the cooking time.
6. When done, the corn and bell peppers should be soft.
7. Transfer them onto a large plate, then spread with feta cheese and cilantro. Drizzle with lemon juice and serve.

481.Simple Air Fried Edamame

Servings:6
Cooking Time: 7 Minutes
Ingredients:
- 1½ pounds (680 g) unshelled edamame
- 2 tablespoons olive oil
- 1 teaspoon sea salt

Directions:
1. Place the edamame in a large bowl, then drizzle with olive oil. Toss to coat well. Transfer the edamame to the air fryer basket.
2. Put the air fryer basket on the baking pan and slide into Rack Position 2, select Air Fry, set temperature to 400ºF (205ºC) and set time to 7 minutes.
3. Stir the edamame at least three times during cooking.
4. When done, the edamame will be tender and warmed through.
5. Transfer the cooked edamame onto a plate and sprinkle with salt. Toss to combine well and set aside for 3 minutes to infuse before serving.

482.Corn On The Cob With Mayonnaise

Servings:4
Cooking Time: 10 Minutes
Ingredients:
- 2 tablespoons mayonnaise
- 2 teaspoons minced garlic
- ½ teaspoon sea salt
- 1 cup panko bread crumbs
- 4 (4-inch length) ears corn on the cob, husk and silk removed
- Cooking spray

Directions:
1. Spritz the air fryer basket with cooking spray.
2. Combine the mayonnaise, garlic, and salt in a bowl. Stir to mix well. Pour the panko on a plate.
3. Brush the corn on the cob with mayonnaise mixture, then roll the cob in the bread crumbs and press to coat well.
4. Transfer the corn on the cob in the basket and spritz with cooking spray.
5. Put the air fryer basket on the baking pan and slide into Rack Position 2, select Air Fry,

set temperature to 400ºF (205ºC) and set time to 10 minutes.

6. Flip the corn on the cob at least three times during the cooking.
7. When cooked, the corn kernels on the cob should be almost browned. Remove from the oven and serve immediately.

483.Lemony Shishito Peppers

Servings:4
Cooking Time: 5 Minutes
Ingredients:
- ½ pound (227 g) shishito peppers (about 24)
- 1 tablespoon olive oil
- Coarse sea salt, to taste
- Lemon wedges, for serving
- Cooking spray

Directions:
1. Spritz the air fryer basket with cooking spray.
2. Toss the peppers with olive oil in a large bowl to coat well.
3. Arrange the peppers in the basket.
4. Put the air fryer basket on the baking pan and slide into Rack Position 2, select Air Fry, set temperature to 400ºF (205ºC) and set time to 5 minutes.
5. Flip the peppers and sprinkle the peppers with salt halfway through the cooking time.
6. When cooked, the peppers should be blistered and lightly charred. Transfer the peppers onto a plate and squeeze the lemon wedges on top before serving.

484.Simple Air Fried Okra Chips

Servings:6
Cooking Time: 16 Minutes
Ingredients:
- 2 pounds (907 g) fresh okra pods, cut into 1-inch pieces
- 2 tablespoons canola oil
- 1 teaspoon coarse sea salt

Directions:
1. Stir the oil and salt in a bowl to mix well. Add the okra and toss to coat well. Place the okra in the air fryer basket.
2. Put the air fryer basket on the baking pan and slide into Rack Position 2, select Air Fry, set temperature to 400ºF (205ºC) and set time to 16 minutes.
3. Flip the okra at least three times during cooking.
4. When cooked, the okra should be lightly browned. Remove from the oven and serve immediately.

485.Sumptuous Beef And Bean Chili Casserole

Servings:4
Cooking Time: 31 Minutes
Ingredients:
- 1 tablespoon olive oil
- ½ cup finely chopped bell pepper
- ½ cup chopped celery
- 1 onion, chopped
- 2 garlic cloves, minced
- 1 pound (454 g) ground beef
- 1 can diced tomatoes
- ½ teaspoon parsley
- ½ tablespoon chili powder
- 1 teaspoon chopped cilantro
- 1½ cups vegetable broth
- 1 (8-ounce / 227-g) can cannellini beans
- Salt and ground black pepper, to taste

Directions:
1. Heat the olive oil in a nonstick skillet over medium heat until shimmering.
2. Add the bell pepper, celery, onion, and garlic to the skillet and sauté for 5 minutes or until the onion is translucent.
3. Add the ground beef and sauté for an additional 6 minutes or until lightly browned.
4. Mix in the tomatoes, parsley, chili powder, cilantro and vegetable broth, then cook for 10 more minutes. Stir constantly.
5. Pour them in the baking pan, then mix in the beans and sprinkle with salt and ground black pepper.
6. Slide the baking pan into Rack Position 1, select Convection Bake, set temperature to 350ºF (180ºC) and set time to 10 minutes.
7. When cooking is complete, the vegetables should be tender and the beef should be well browned.
8. Remove from the oven and serve immediately.

486.Lush Seafood Casserole

Servings:2
Cooking Time: 22 Minutes
Ingredients:
- 1 tablespoon olive oil
- 1 small yellow onion, chopped
- 2 garlic cloves, minced
- 4 ounces (113 g) tilapia pieces
- 4 ounces (113 g) rockfish pieces
- ½ teaspoon dried basil
- Salt and ground white pepper, to taste
- 4 eggs, lightly beaten
- 1 tablespoon dry sherry
- 4 tablespoons cheese, shredded

Directions:

1. Heat the olive oil in a nonstick skillet over medium-high heat until shimmering.
2. Add the onion and garlic and sauté for 2 minutes or until fragrant.
3. Add the tilapia, rockfish, basil, salt, and white pepper to the skillet. Sauté to combine well and transfer them into the baking pan.
4. Combine the eggs, sherry and cheese in a large bowl. Stir to mix well. Pour the mixture in the baking pan over the fish mixture.
5. Slide the baking pan into Rack Position 1, select Convection Bake, set temperature to 360ºF (182ºC) and set time to 20 minutes.
6. When cooking is complete, the eggs should be set and the casserole edges should be lightly browned.
7. Serve immediately.

487.Air Fried Bacon Pinwheels

Servings: 8 Pinwheels
Cooking Time: 10 Minutes
Ingredients:
- 1 sheet puff pastry
- 2 tablespoons maple syrup
- ¼ cup brown sugar
- 8 slices bacon
- Ground black pepper, to taste
- Cooking spray

Directions:
1. Spritz the air fryer basket with cooking spray.
2. Roll the puff pastry into a 10-inch square with a rolling pin on a clean work surface, then cut the pastry into 8 strips.
3. Brush the strips with maple syrup and sprinkle with sugar, leaving a 1-inch far end uncovered.
4. Arrange each slice of bacon on each strip, leaving a ⅛-inch length of bacon hang over the end close to you. Sprinkle with black pepper.
5. From the end close to you, roll the strips into pinwheels, then dab the uncovered end with water and seal the rolls.
6. Arrange the pinwheels in the basket and spritz with cooking spray.
7. Put the air fryer basket on the baking pan and slide into Rack Position 2, select Air Fry, set temperature to 360ºF (182ºC) and set time to 10 minutes.
8. Flip the pinwheels halfway through.
9. When cooking is complete, the pinwheels should be golden brown. Remove from the oven and serve immediately.

488.Parsnip Fries With Garlic-yogurt Dip

Servings:4
Cooking Time: 10 Minutes

Ingredients:
- 3 medium parsnips, peeled, cut into sticks
- ¼ teaspoon kosher salt
- 1 teaspoon olive oil
- 1 garlic clove, unpeeled
- Cooking spray
- Dip:
- ¼ cup plain Greek yogurt
- ⅛ teaspoon garlic powder
- 1 tablespoon sour cream
- ¼ teaspoon kosher salt
- Freshly ground black pepper, to taste

Directions:
1. Spritz the air fryer basket with cooking spray.
2. Put the parsnip sticks in a large bowl, then sprinkle with salt and drizzle with olive oil.
3. Transfer the parsnip into the basket and add the garlic.
4. Put the air fryer basket on the baking pan and slide into Rack Position 2, select Air Fry, set temperature to 360ºF (182ºC) and set time to 10 minutes.
5. Stir the parsnip halfway through the cooking time.
6. Meanwhile, peel the garlic and crush it. Combine the crushed garlic with the ingredients for the dip. Stir to mix well.
7. When cooked, the parsnip sticks should be crisp. Remove the parsnip fries from the oven and serve with the dipping sauce.

489. Citrus Avocado Wedge Fries

Servings: 12 Fries
Cooking Time: 8 Minutes
Ingredients:
- 1 cup all-purpose flour
- 3 tablespoons lime juice
- ¾ cup orange juice
- 1¼ cups plain dried bread crumbs
- 1 cup yellow cornmeal
- 1½ tablespoons chile powder
- 2 large Hass avocados, peeled, pitted, and cut into wedges
- Coarse sea salt, to taste
- Cooking spray

Directions:
1. Spritz the air fryer basket with cooking spray.
2. Pour the flour in a bowl. Mix the lime juice with orange juice in a second bowl. Combine the bread crumbs, cornmeal, and chile powder in a third bowl.
3. Dip the avocado wedges in the bowl of flour to coat well, then dredge the wedges into the bowl of juice mixture, and then dunk the wedges in the bread crumbs mixture. Shake the excess off.

4. Arrange the coated avocado wedges in a single layer in the basket. Spritz with cooking spray.
5. Put the air fryer basket on the baking pan and slide into Rack Position 2, select Air Fry, set temperature to 400ºF (205ºC) and set time to 8 minutes.
6. Stir the avocado wedges and sprinkle with salt halfway through the cooking time.
7. When cooking is complete, the avocado wedges should be tender and crispy.
8. Serve immediately.

490. Traditional Latkes

Servings: 4 Latkes
Cooking Time: 10 Minutes
Ingredients:
- 1 egg
- 2 tablespoons all-purpose flour
- 2 medium potatoes, peeled and shredded, rinsed and drained
- ¼ teaspoon granulated garlic
- ½ teaspoon salt
- Cooking spray

Directions:
1. Spritz the air fryer basket with cooking spray.
2. Whisk together the egg, flour, potatoes, garlic, and salt in a large bowl. Stir to mix well.
3. Divide the mixture into four parts, then flatten them into four circles. Arrange the circles onto the basket and spritz with cooking spray.
4. Put the air fryer basket on the baking pan and slide into Rack Position 2, select Air Fry, set temperature to 380ºF (193ºC) and set time to 10 minutes.
5. Flip the latkes halfway through.
6. When cooked, the latkes will be golden brown and crispy. Remove from the oven and serve immediately.

491. Arancini

Servings: 10 Arancini
Cooking Time: 30 Minutes
Ingredients:
- ²/₃ cup raw white Arborio rice
- 2 teaspoons butter
- ½ teaspoon salt
- 1¹/₃ cups water
- 2 large eggs, well beaten
- 1¼ cups seasoned Italian-style dried bread crumbs
- 10 ¾-inch semi-firm Mozzarella cubes
- Cooking spray

Directions:

1. Pour the rice, butter, salt, and water in a pot. Stir to mix well and bring a boil over medium-high heat. Keep stirring.
2. Reduce the heat to low and cover the pot. Simmer for 20 minutes or until the rice is tender.
3. Turn off the heat and let sit, covered, for 10 minutes, then open the lid and fluffy the rice with a fork. Allow to cool for 10 more minutes.
4. Pour the beaten eggs in a bowl, then pour the bread crumbs in a separate bowl.
5. Scoop 2 tablespoons of the cooked rice up and form it into a ball, then press the Mozzarella into the ball and wrap.
6. Dredge the ball in the eggs first, then shake the excess off the dunk the ball in the bread crumbs. Roll to coat evenly. Repeat to make 10 balls in total with remaining rice.
7. Transfer the balls in the air fryer basket and spritz with cooking spray.
8. Put the air fryer basket on the baking pan and slide into Rack Position 2, select Air Fry, set temperature to 375ºF (190ºC) and set time to 10 minutes.
9. When cooking is complete, the balls should be lightly browned and crispy.
10. Remove the balls from the oven and allow to cool before serving.

492.Roasted Mushrooms

Servings: About 1½ Cups
Cooking Time: 30 Minutes
Ingredients:
- 1 pound (454 g) button or cremini mushrooms, washed, stems trimmed, and cut into quarters or thick slices
- ¼ cup water
- 1 teaspoon kosher salt or ½ teaspoon fine salt
- 3 tablespoons unsalted butter, cut into pieces, or extra-virgin olive oil

Directions:
1. Place a large piece of aluminum foil on the sheet pan. Place the mushroom pieces in the middle of the foil. Spread them out into an even layer. Pour the water over them, season with the salt, and add the butter. Wrap the mushrooms in the foil.
2. Select Roast, set the temperature to 325ºF (163ºC), and set the time for 15 minutes. Select Start to begin preheating.
3. Once the unit has preheated, place the pan in the oven.
4. After 15 minutes, remove the pan from the oven. Transfer the foil packet to a cutting board and carefully unwrap it. Pour the mushrooms and cooking liquid from the foil onto the sheet pan.

5. Select Roast, set the temperature to 350ºF (180ºC), and set the time for 15 minutes. Return the pan to the oven. Select Start to begin.
6. After about 10 minutes, remove the pan from the oven and stir the mushrooms. Return the pan to the oven and continue cooking for anywhere from 5 to 15 more minutes, or until the liquid is mostly gone and the mushrooms start to brown.
7. Serve immediately.

493.Air Fried Crispy Brussels Sprouts

Servings:4
Cooking Time: 20 Minutes
Ingredients:
- ¼ teaspoon salt
- ⅛ teaspoon ground black pepper
- 1 tablespoon extra-virgin olive oil
- 1 pound (454 g) Brussels sprouts, trimmed and halved
- Lemon wedges, for garnish

Directions:
1. Combine the salt, black pepper, and olive oil in a large bowl. Stir to mix well.
2. Add the Brussels sprouts to the bowl of mixture and toss to coat well. Arrange the Brussels sprouts in the air fryer basket.
3. Put the air fryer basket on the baking pan and slide into Rack Position 2, select Air Fry, set temperature to 350ºF (180ºC) and set time to 20 minutes.
4. Stir the Brussels sprouts two times during cooking.
5. When cooked, the Brussels sprouts will be lightly browned and wilted. Transfer the cooked Brussels sprouts to a large plate and squeeze the lemon wedges on top to serve.

494.Supplì Al Telefono (risotto Croquettes)

Servings:6
Cooking Time: 54 Minutes
Ingredients:
- Risotto Croquettes:
- 4 tablespoons unsalted butter
- 1 small yellow onion, minced
- 1 cup Arborio rice
- 3½ cups chicken stock
- ½ cup dry white wine
- 3 eggs
- Zest of 1 lemon
- ½ cup grated Parmesan cheese
- 2 ounces (57 g) fresh Mozzarella cheese
- ¼ cup peas
- 2 tablespoons water
- ½ cup all-purpose flour
- 1½ cups panko bread crumbs

- Kosher salt and ground black pepper, to taste
- Cooking spray
- Tomato Sauce:
- 2 tablespoons extra-virgin olive oil
- 4 cloves garlic, minced
- ¼ teaspoon red pepper flakes
- 1 (28-ounce / 794-g) can crushed tomatoes
- 2 teaspoons granulated sugar
- Kosher salt and ground black pepper, to taste

Directions:
1. Melt the butter in a pot over medium heat, then add the onion and salt to taste. Sauté for 5 minutes or until the onion in translucent.
2. Add the rice and stir to coat well. Cook for 3 minutes or until the rice is lightly browned. Pour in the chicken stock and wine.
3. Bring to a boil. Then cook for 20 minutes or until the rice is tender and liquid is almost absorbed.
4. Make the risotto: When the rice is cooked, break the egg into the pot. Add the lemon zest and Parmesan cheese. Sprinkle with salt and ground black pepper. Stir to mix well.
5. Pour the risotto in a baking sheet, then level with a spatula to spread the risotto evenly. Wrap the baking sheet in plastic and refrigerate for1 hour.
6. Meanwhile, heat the olive oil in a saucepan over medium heat until shimmering.
7. Add the garlic and sprinkle with red pepper flakes. Sauté for a minute or until fragrant.
8. Add the crushed tomatoes and sprinkle with sugar. Stir to mix well. Bring to a boil. Reduce the heat to low and simmer for 15 minutes or until lightly thickened. Sprinkle with salt and pepper to taste. Set aside until ready to serve.
9. Remove the risotto from the refrigerator. Scoop the risotto into twelve 2-inch balls, then flatten the balls with your hands.
10. Arrange a about ½-inch piece of Mozzarella and 5 peas in the center of each flattened ball, then wrap them back into balls.
11. Transfer the balls to a baking sheet lined with parchment paper, then refrigerate for 15 minutes or until firm.
12. Whisk the remaining 2 eggs with 2 tablespoons of water in a bowl. Pour the flour in a second bowl and pour the panko in a third bowl.
13. Dredge the risotto balls in the bowl of flour first, then into the eggs, and then into the panko. Shake the excess off.
14. Transfer the balls to the baking pan and spritz with cooking spray.
15. Slide the baking pan into Rack Position 1, select Convection Bake, set temperature to 400ºF (205ºC) and set time to 10 minutes.
16. Flip the balls halfway through the cooking time.
17. When cooking is complete, the balls should be until golden brown.
18. Serve the risotto balls with the tomato sauce.

495.Burgundy Beef And Mushroom Casserole

Servings:4
Cooking Time: 25 Minutes
Ingredients:
- 1½ pounds (680 g) beef steak
- 1 ounce (28 g) dry onion soup mix
- 2 cups sliced mushrooms
- 1 (14.5-ounce / 411-g) can cream of mushroom soup
- ½ cup beef broth
- ¼ cup red wine
- 3 garlic cloves, minced
- 1 whole onion, chopped

Directions:
1. Put the beef steak in a large bowl, then sprinkle with dry onion soup mix. Toss to coat well.
2. Combine the mushrooms with mushroom soup, beef broth, red wine, garlic, and onion in a large bowl. Stir to mix well.
3. Transfer the beef steak in the baking pan, then pour in the mushroom mixture.
4. Slide the baking pan into Rack Position 1, select Convection Bake, set temperature to 360ºF (182ºC) and set time to 25 minutes.
5. When cooking is complete, the mushrooms should be soft and the beef should be well browned.
6. Remove from the oven and serve immediately.

496.Sweet Cinnamon Chickpeas

Servings:2
Cooking Time: 10 Minutes
Ingredients:
- 1 tablespoon cinnamon
- 1 tablespoon sugar
- 1 cup chickpeas, soaked in water overnight, rinsed and drained

Directions:
1. Combine the cinnamon and sugar in a bowl. Stir to mix well.
2. Add the chickpeas to the bowl, then toss to coat well.
3. Pour the chickpeas in the air fryer basket.
4. Put the air fryer basket on the baking pan and slide into Rack Position 2, select Air Fry,

set temperature to 390ºF (199ºC) and set time to 10 minutes.

5. Stir the chickpeas three times during cooking.
6. When cooked, the chickpeas should be golden brown and crispy. Remove from the oven and serve immediately.

497.Classic Churros

Servings: 12 Churros
Cooking Time: 10 Minutes
Ingredients:
- 4 tablespoons butter
- ¼ teaspoon salt
- ½ cup water
- ½ cup all-purpose flour
- 2 large eggs
- 2 teaspoons ground cinnamon
- ¼ cup granulated white sugar
- Cooking spray

Directions:
1. Put the butter, salt, and water in a saucepan. Bring to a boil until the butter is melted on high heat. Keep stirring.
2. Reduce the heat to medium and fold in the flour to form a dough. Keep cooking and stirring until the dough is dried out and coat the pan with a crust.
3. Turn off the heat and scrape the dough in a large bowl. Allow to cool for 15 minutes.
4. Break and whisk the eggs into the dough with a hand mixer until the dough is sanity and firm enough to shape.
5. Scoop up 1 tablespoon of the dough and roll it into a ½-inch-diameter and 2-inch-long cylinder. Repeat with remaining dough to make 12 cylinders in total.
6. Combine the cinnamon and sugar in a large bowl and dunk the cylinders into the cinnamon mix to coat.
7. Arrange the cylinders on a plate and refrigerate for 20 minutes.
8. Spritz the air fryer basket with cooking spray. Place the cylinders in the basket and spritz with cooking spray.
9. Put the air fryer basket on the baking pan and slide into Rack Position 2, select Air Fry, set temperature to 375ºF (190ºC) and set time to 10 minutes.
10. Flip the cylinders halfway through the cooking time.
11. When cooked, the cylinders should be golden brown and fluffy.
12. Serve immediately.

498.Dehydrated Crackers With Oats

Servings:x
Cooking Time:x
Ingredients:
- 3 tablespoons (20g) psyllium husk powder
- 2 teaspoons fine sea salt
- 1 teaspoon freshly ground black pepper
- 2 teaspoons ground turmeric, divided
- 3 tablespoons melted coconut oil
- 1 cup (125g) sunflower seeds
- ½ cup (75g) flaxseeds
- ¾ cup (50g) pumpkin seeds
- ¼ cup (35g) sesame seeds
- 2 tablespoons (30g) chia seeds
- 1½ cups (150g) rolled oats
- 1½ cups (360ml) water
- 1 large parsnip (10 ounces/300g), finely Grated

Directions:
1. In a large bowl Blend All of the seeds, Oats, psyllium husk, pepper, salt and 1 teaspoon ground turmeric.
2. Whisk coconut water and oil together in a measuring Cup. Add to the dry ingredients and blend well until all is totally saturated and dough becomes very thick.
3. Mix grated parsnip using 1 tsp turmeric and stir to blend.
4. Shape the first half to a disc and place it with a rolling pin, firmly roll dough to a thin sheet that the size of this dehydrate basket.
5. Put dough and parchment paper at the dehydrate basket.
6. Repeat steps 4 with remaining dough.
7. Hours and allow Rotate Remind. Place dehydrate baskets in rack positions 5 and 3. Press START.
8. Dehydrate crackers until tender. When prompted By Rotate Remind, rotate the baskets leading to back and change rack amounts.
9. Eliminate baskets out of oven and let rest for 10 minutes. Split crackers into shards.
10. Container for up to two months.

499.Chinese Pork And Mushroom Egg Rolls

Servings: 25 Egg Rolls
Cooking Time: 33 Minutes
Ingredients:
- Egg Rolls:
- 1 tablespoon mirin
- 3 tablespoons soy sauce, divided
- 1 pound (454 g) ground pork
- 3 tablespoons vegetable oil, plus more for brushing
- 5 ounces (142 g) shiitake mushrooms, minced
- 4 cups shredded Napa cabbage
- ¼ cup sliced scallions
- 1 teaspoon grated fresh ginger
- 1 clove garlic, minced
- ¼ teaspoon cornstarch

- 1 (1-pound / 454-g) package frozen egg roll wrappers, thawed
- Dipping Sauce:
- 1 scallion, white and light green parts only, sliced
- ¼ cup rice vinegar
- ¼ cup soy sauce
- Pinch sesame seeds
- Pinch red pepper flakes
- 1 teaspoon granulated sugar

Directions:
1. Line the air fryer basket with parchment paper. Set aside.
2. Combine the mirin and 1 tablespoon of soy sauce in a large bowl. Stir to mix well.
3. Dunk the ground pork in the mixture and stir to mix well. Wrap the bowl in plastic and marinate in the refrigerator for at least 10 minutes.
4. Heat the vegetable oil in a nonstick skillet over medium-high heat until shimmering. Add the mushrooms, cabbage, and scallions and sauté for 5 minutes or until tender.
5. Add the marinated meat, ginger, garlic, and remaining 2 tablespoons of soy sauce. Sauté for 3 minutes or until the pork is lightly browned. Turn off the heat and allow to cool until ready to use.
6. Put the cornstarch in a small bowl and pour in enough water to dissolve the cornstarch. Put the bowl alongside a clean work surface.
7. Put the egg roll wrappers in the basket.
8. Put the air fryer basket on the baking pan and slide into Rack Position 2, select Air Fry, set temperature to 400ºF (205ºC) and set time to 15 minutes.
9. Flip the wrappers halfway through the cooking time.
10. When cooked, the wrappers will be golden brown. Remove the egg roll wrappers from the oven and allow to cool for 10 minutes or until you can handle them with your hands.
11. Lay out one egg roll wrapper on the work surface with a corner pointed toward you. Place 2 tablespoons of the pork mixture on the egg roll wrapper and fold corner up over the mixture. Fold left and right corners toward the center and continue to roll. Brush a bit of the dissolved cornstarch on the last corner to help seal the egg wrapper.

Repeat with remaining wrappers to make 25 egg rolls in total.
12. Arrange the rolls in the basket and brush the rolls with more vegetable oil.
13. Select Air Fry and set time to 10 minutes. Return to the oven. When done, the rolls should be well browned and crispy.
14. Meanwhile, combine the ingredients for the dipping sauce in a small bowl. Stir to mix well.
15. Serve the rolls with the dipping sauce immediately.

500.Dehydrated Honey-rosemary Roasted Almonds

Servings:x
Cooking Time:x
Ingredients:
- 1 heaping tablespoon demerara sugar
- 1 teaspoon finely chopped fresh rosemary
- 1 teaspoon kosher salt
- 8 ounces (225g) raw almonds
- 2 tablespoons kosher salt
- Honey-Rosemary glaze
- ¼ cup (80g) honey

Directions:
1. Place almonds and salt in a bowl. Add cold tap water to cover the almonds by 1-inch
2. (2cm). Let soak at room temperature for 12 hours to activate.
3. Rinse almonds under cold running water, then drain. Spread in a single layer on the dehydrate basket.
4. Dehydrate almonds for 24 hours or till tender and somewhat crispy but additionally spongy in the middle. Almonds may be eaten plain or roasted each the next recipe.
5. Put honey in a small saucepan and heat over Low heat. Put triggered nuts
6. At a medium bowl and then pour over warm honey. Stir To coat nuts equally. Add rosemary, sugar
7. And salt and stir to blend.
8. Spread Almonds in one layer on the skillet.
9. Insert cable rack into rack place 6. Select BAKE/350°F (175°C)/CONVECTION/10 moments and empower Rotate Remind.
10. Stirring almonds when Rotate Remind signs.
11. Let cool completely before storing in an airtight container.

CPSIA information can be obtained
at www.ICGtesting.com
Printed in the USA
LVHW010514260121
677404LV00009B/596